#STAY HOME

Pete Slater

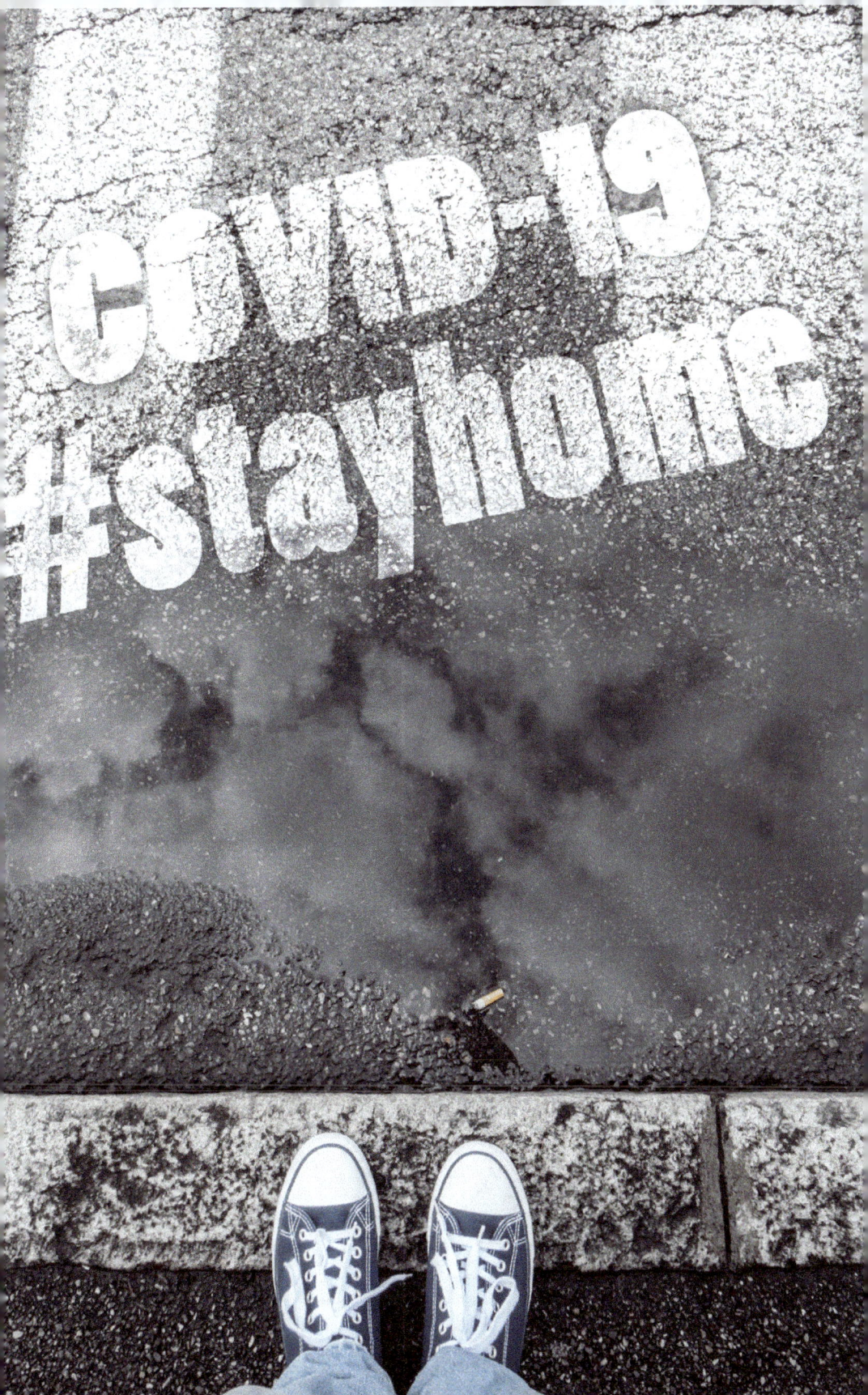

the great equalizer.

Madonna

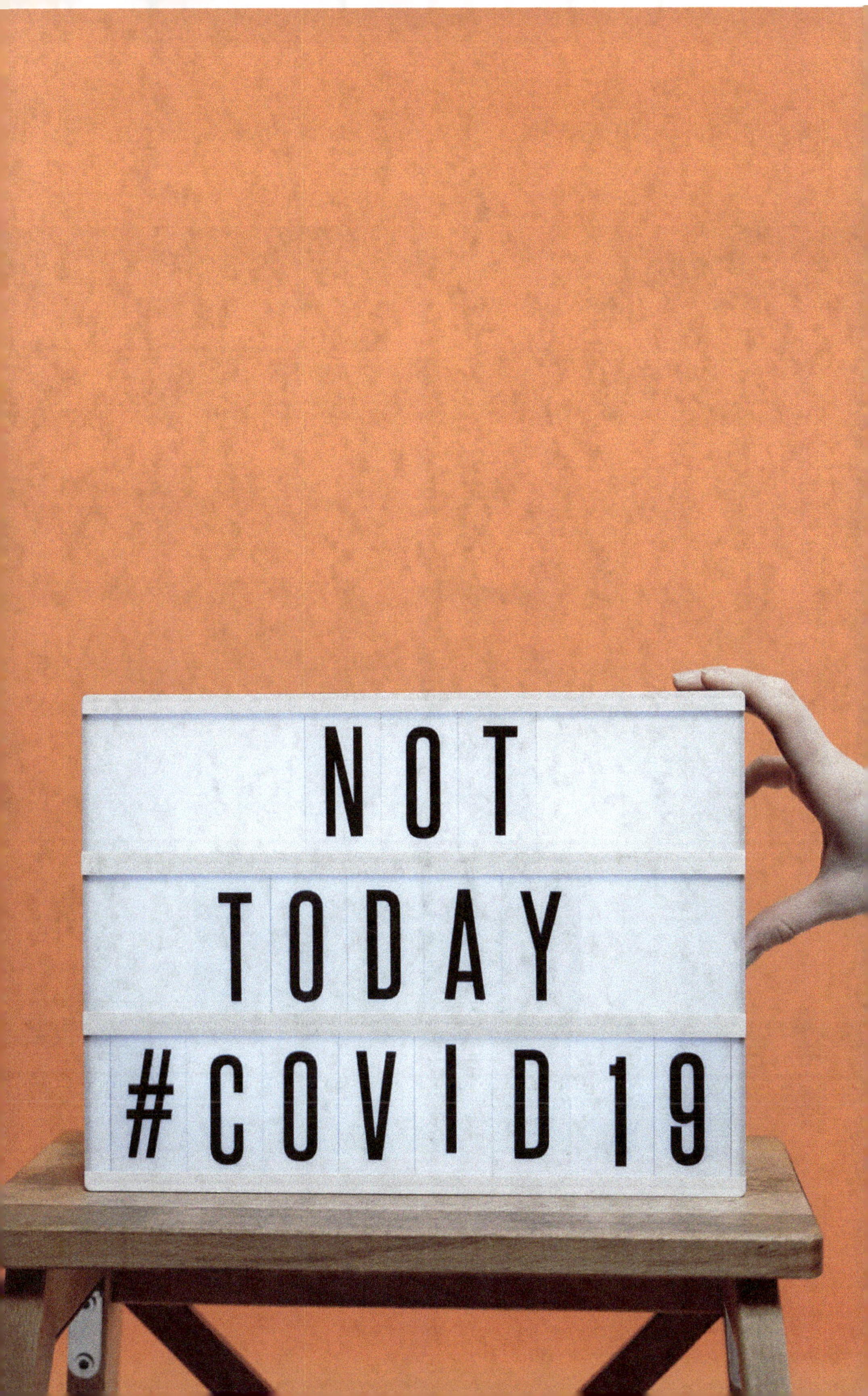
NOT
TODAY
#COVID19

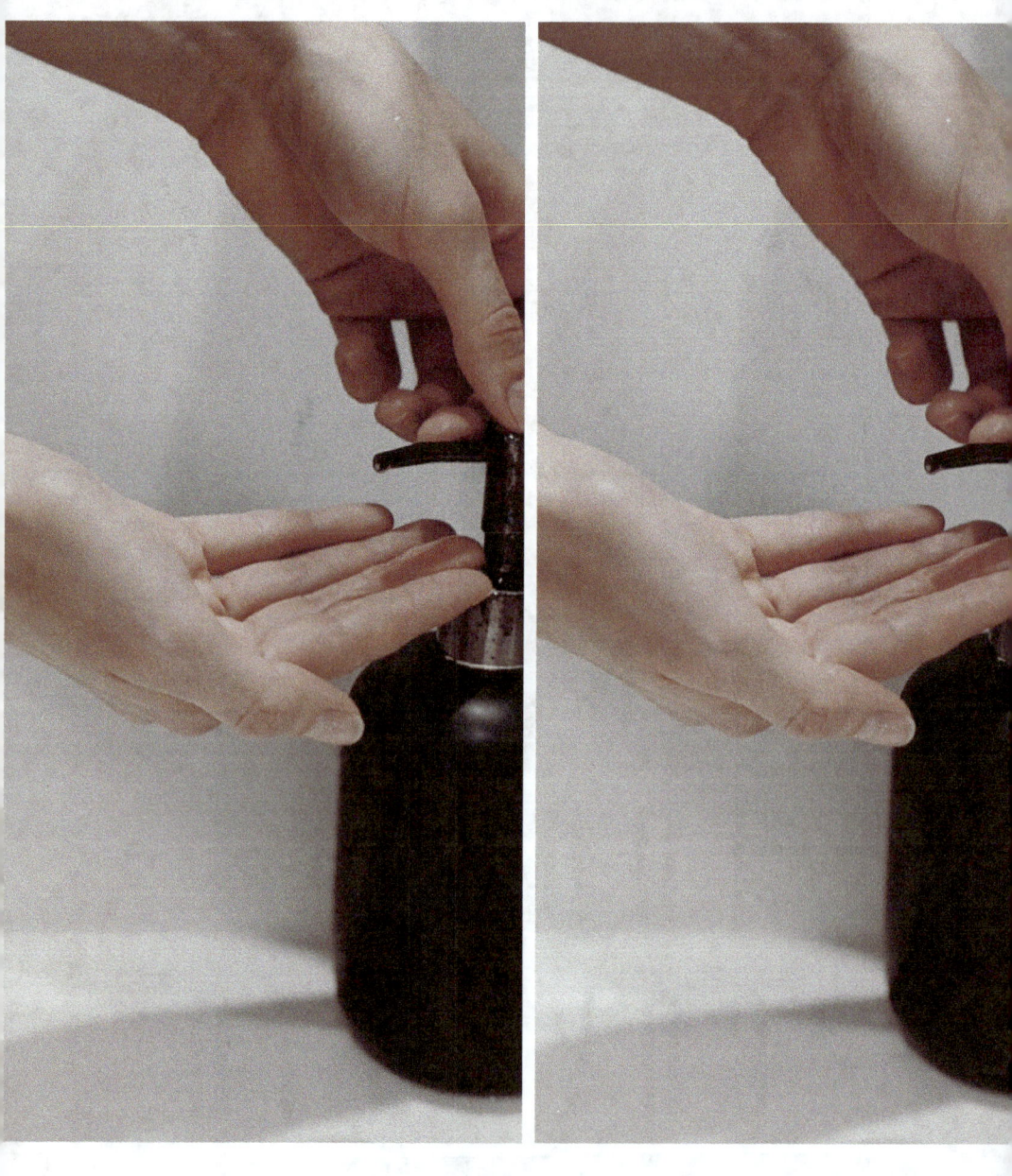

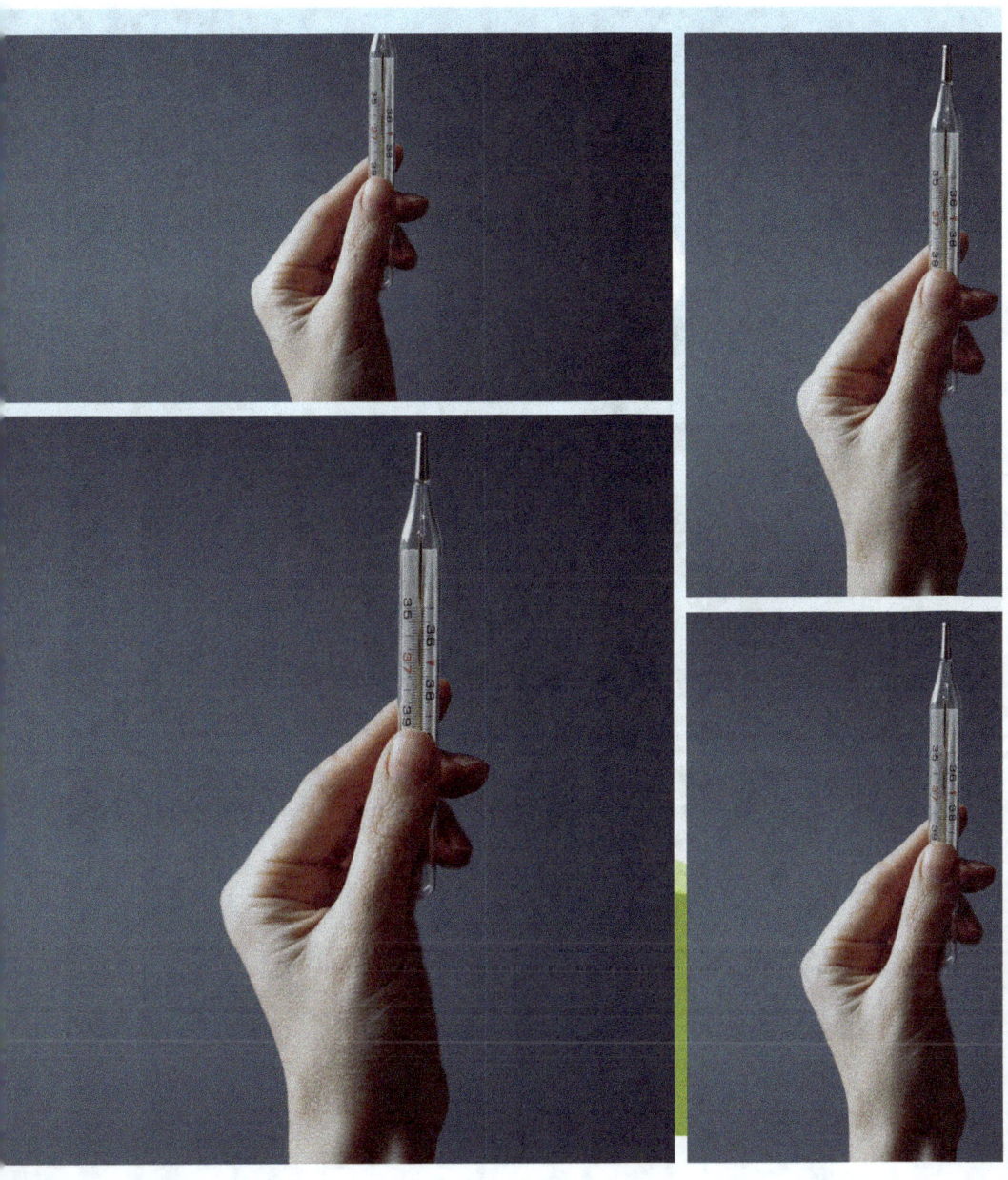

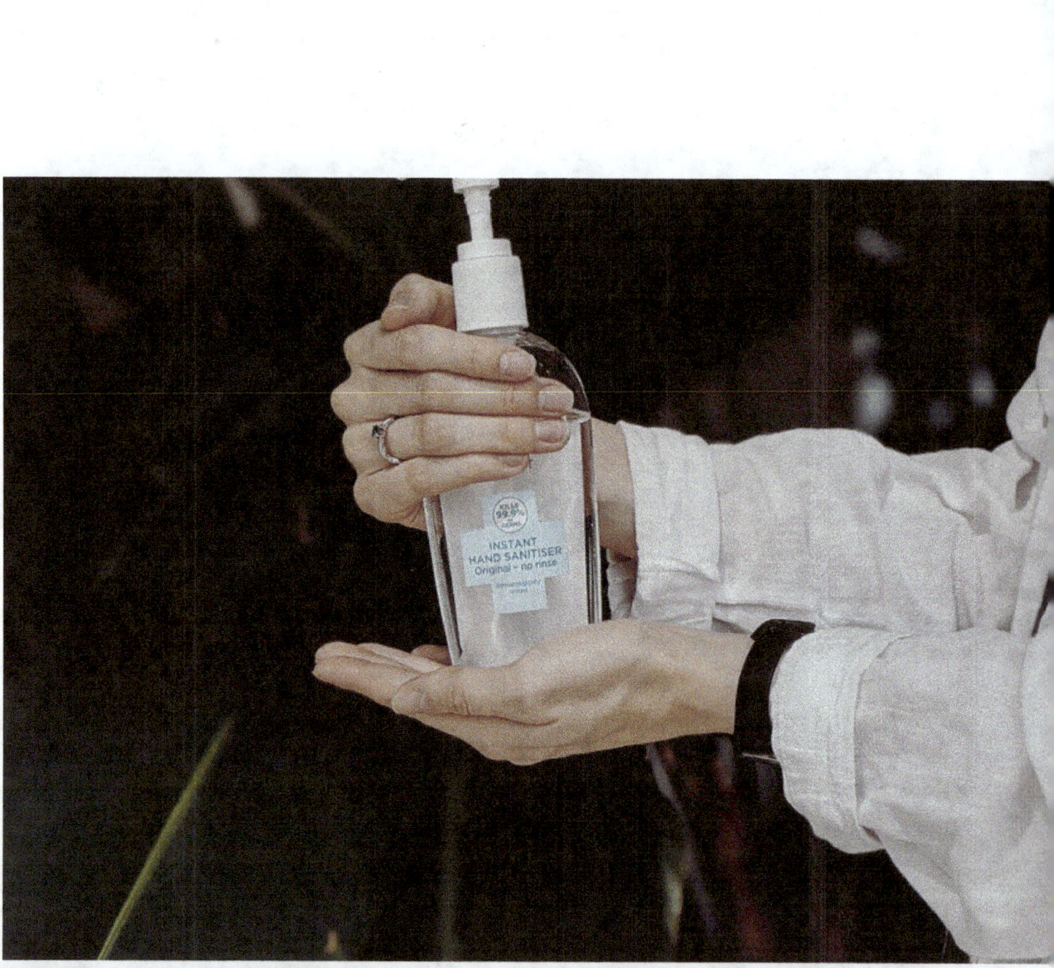

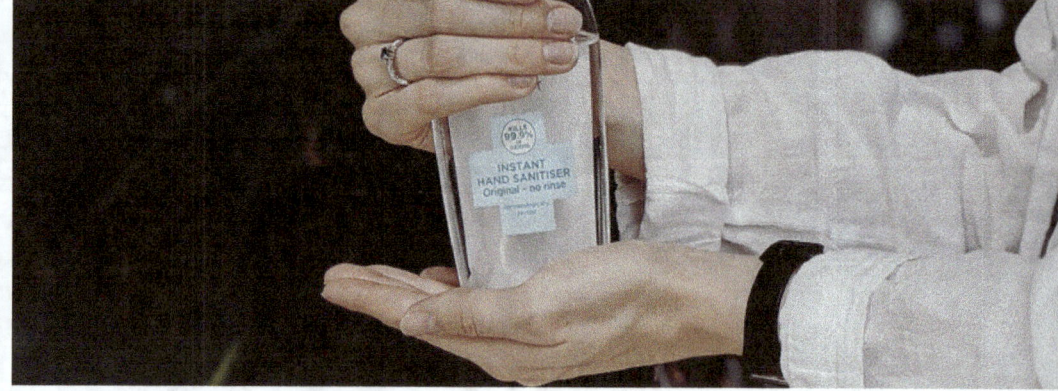

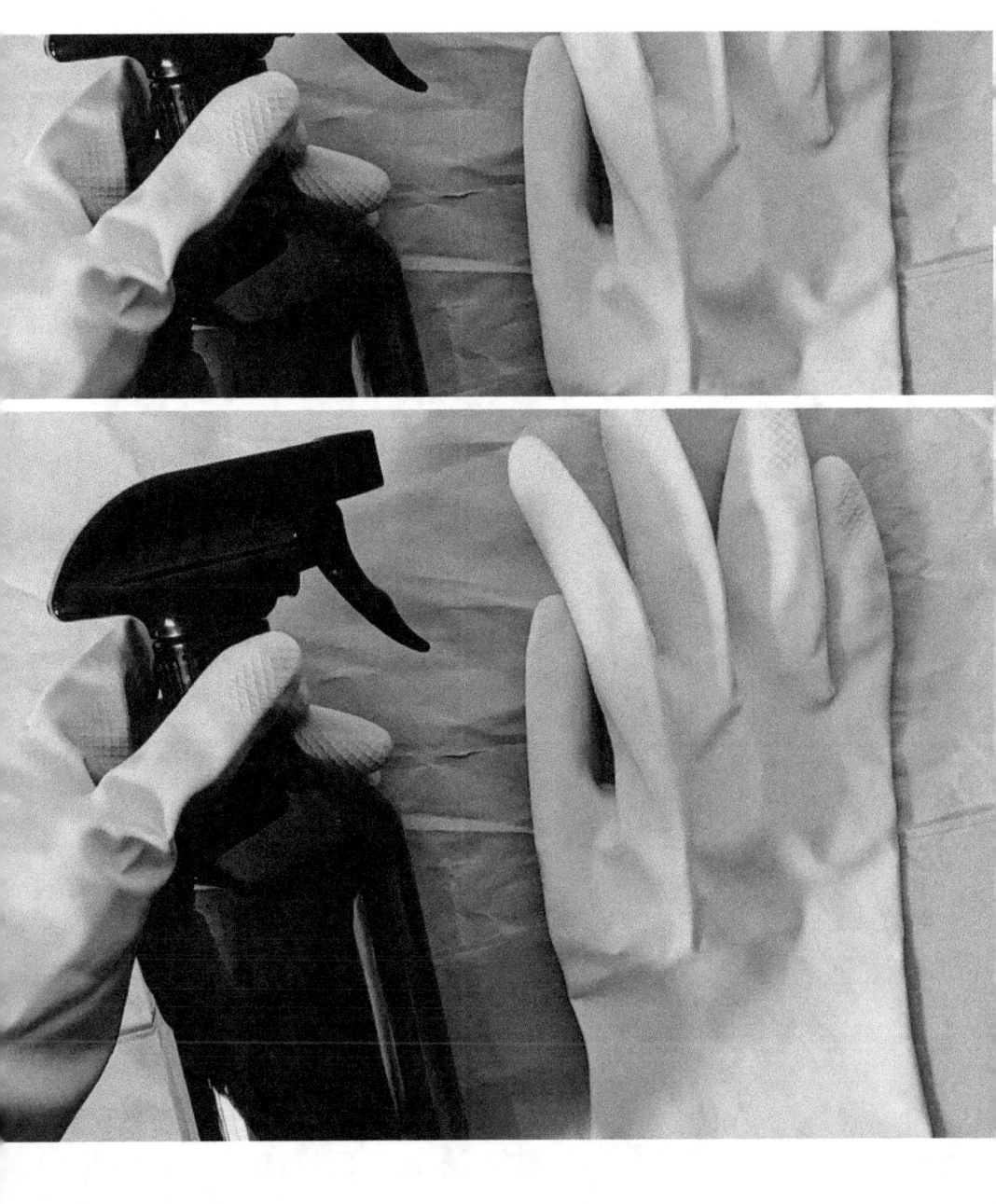

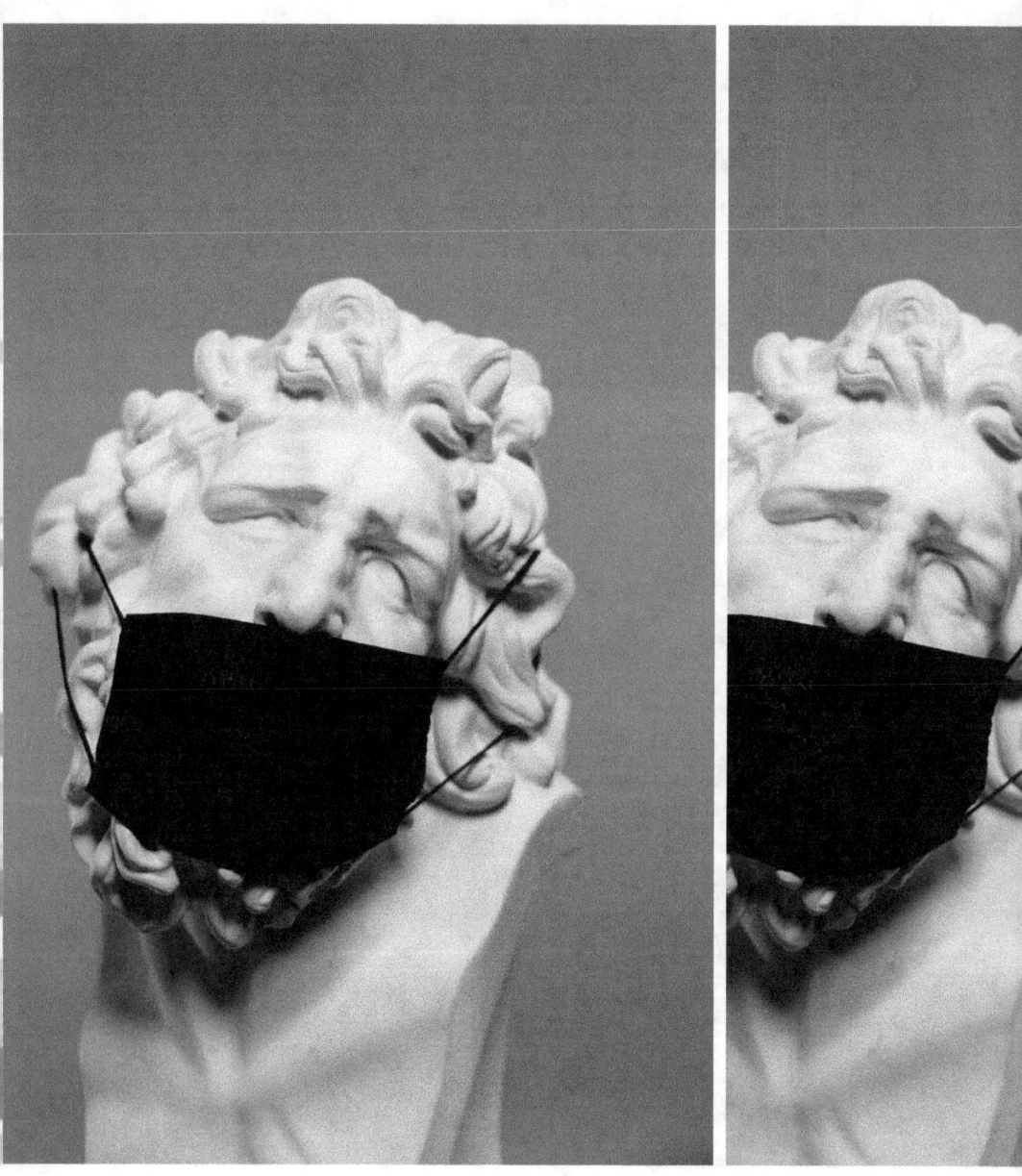

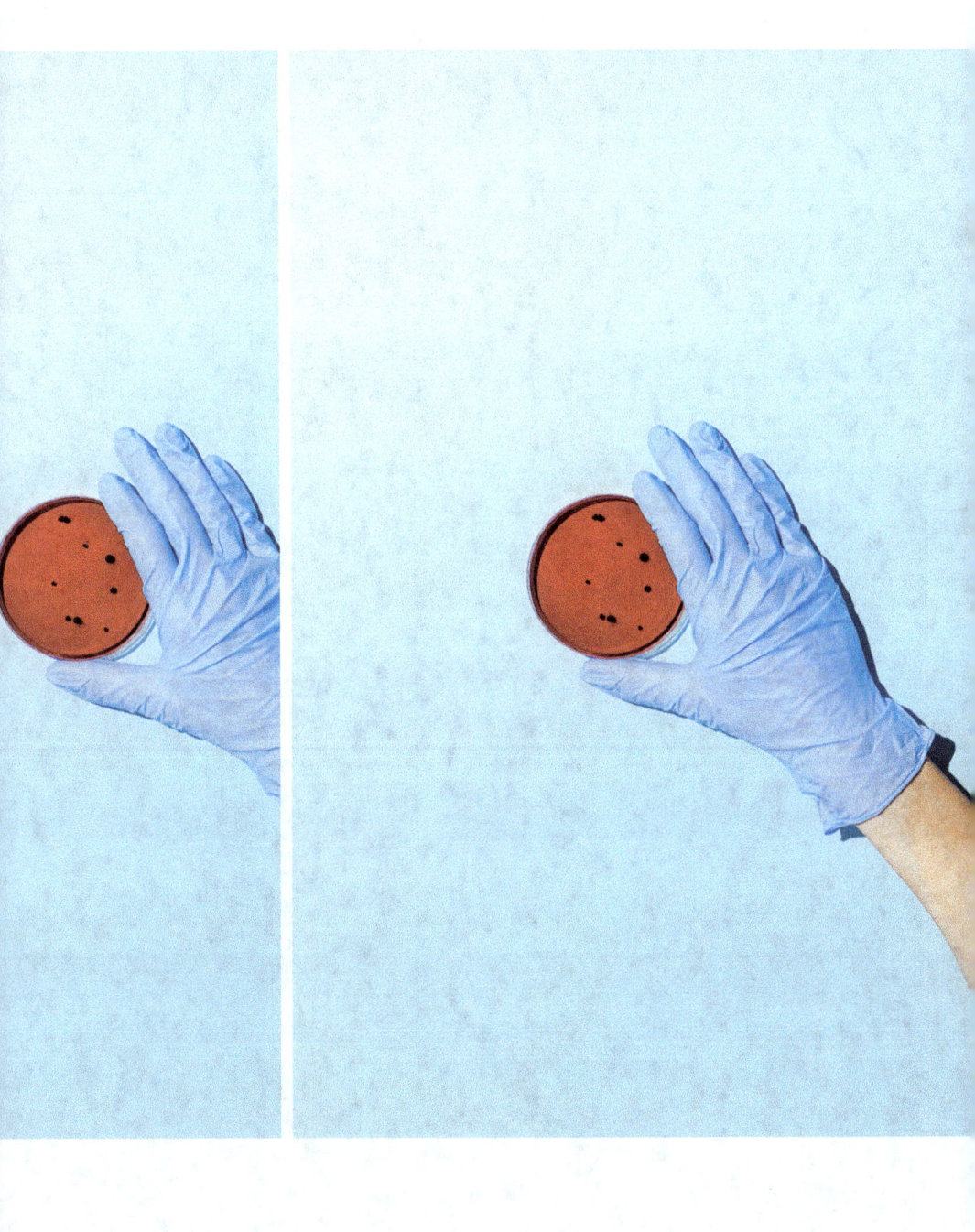

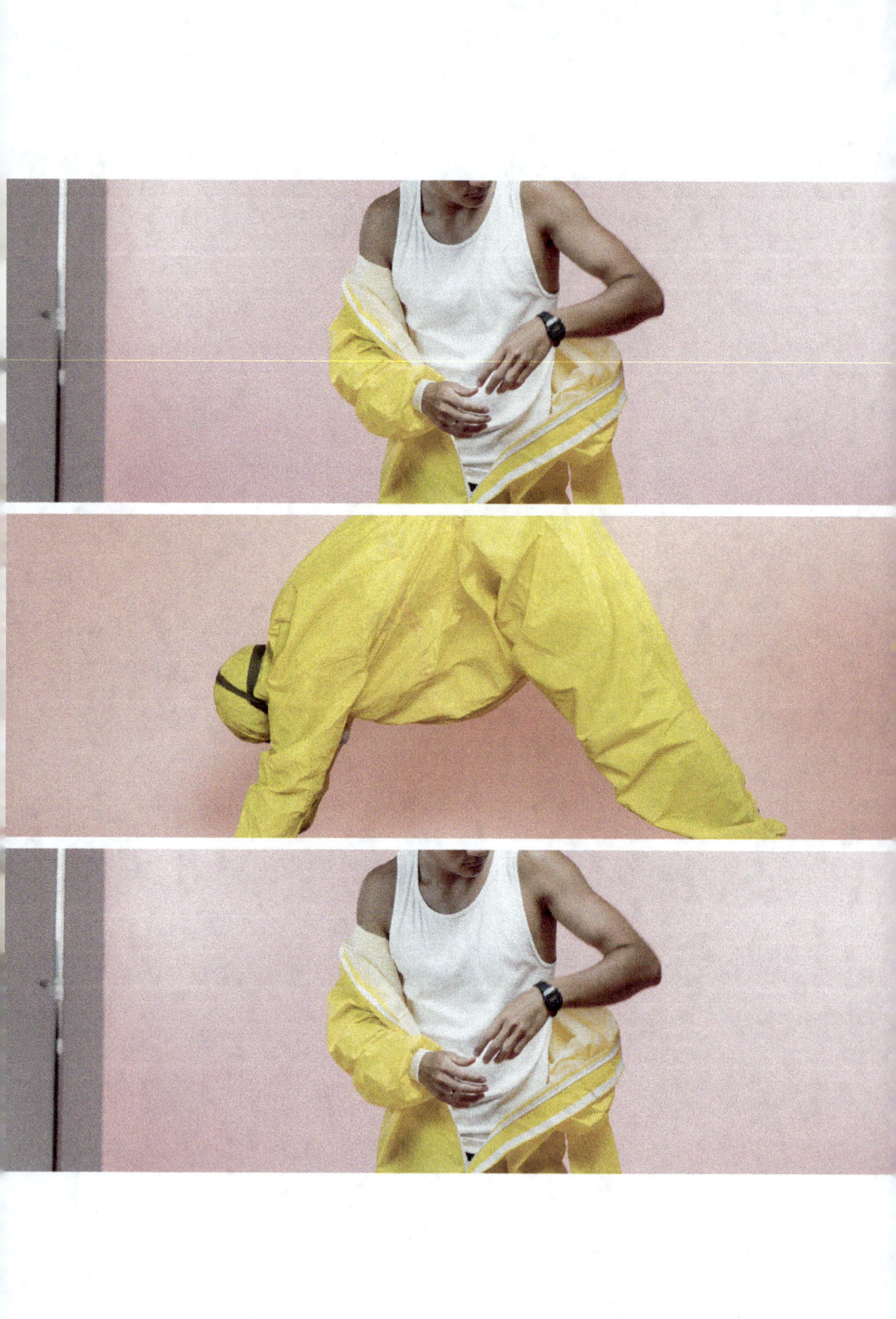

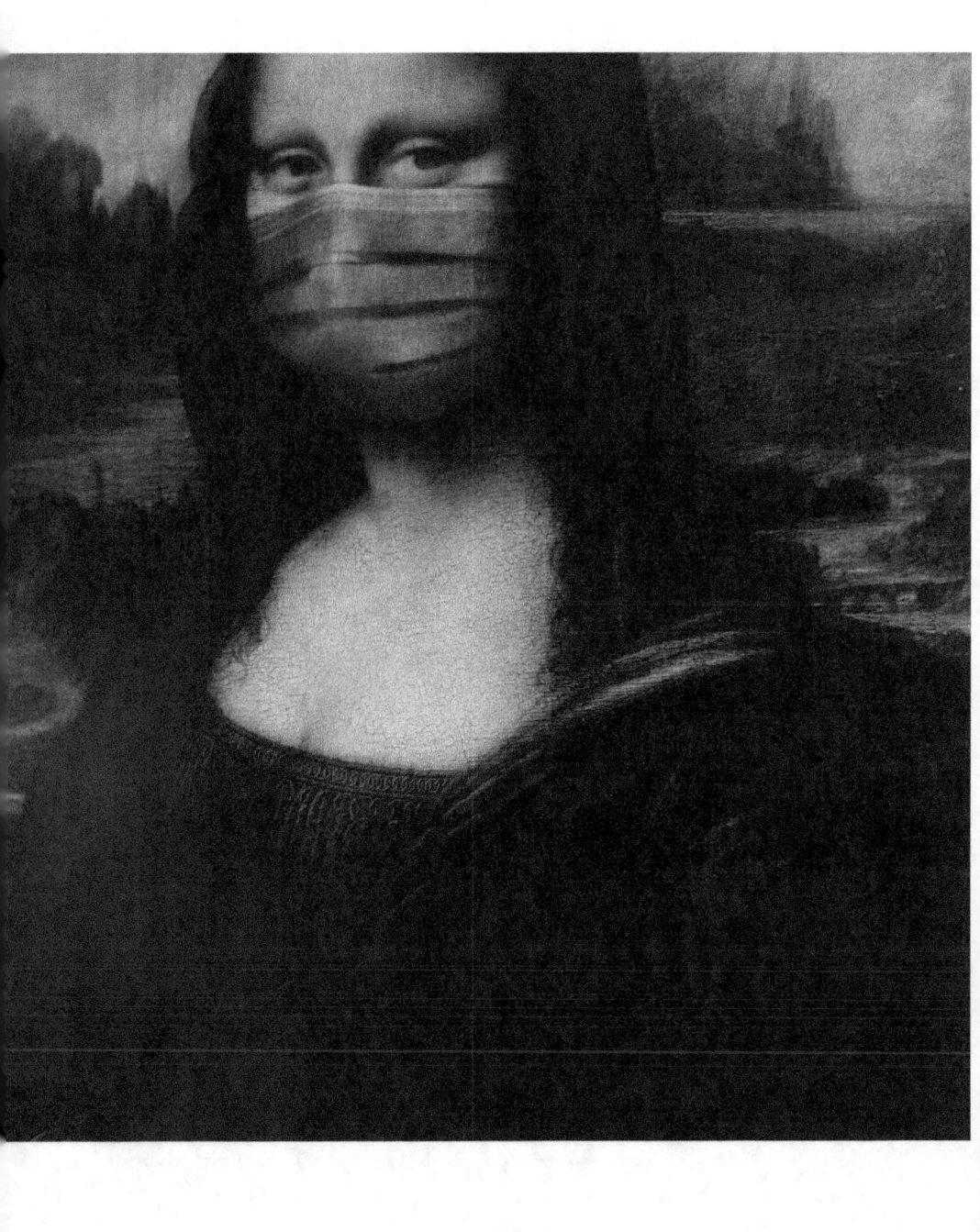

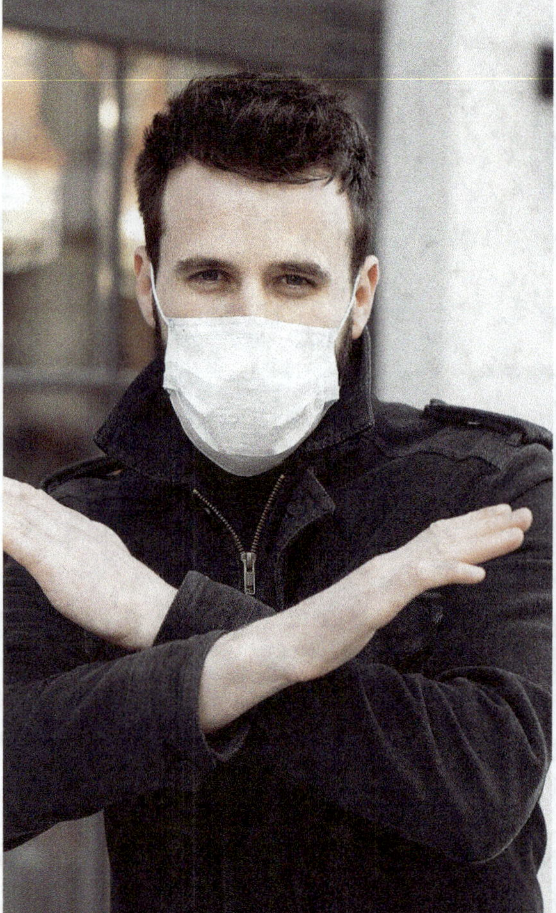

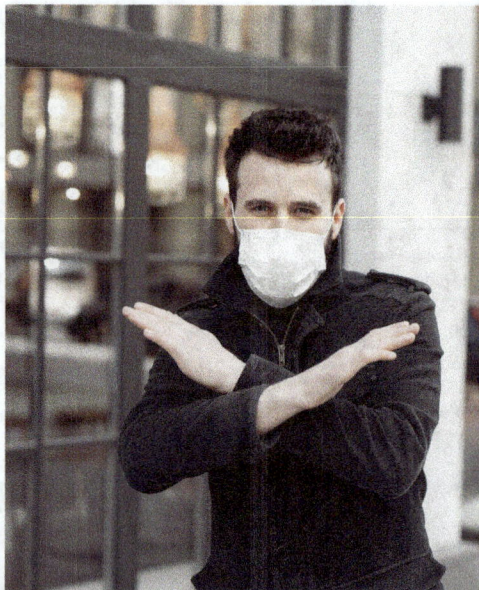
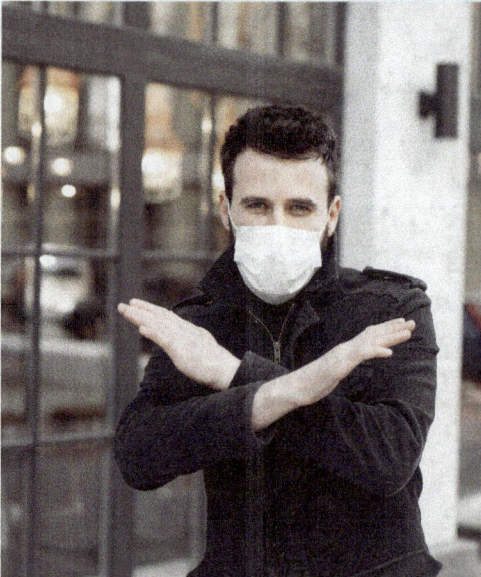

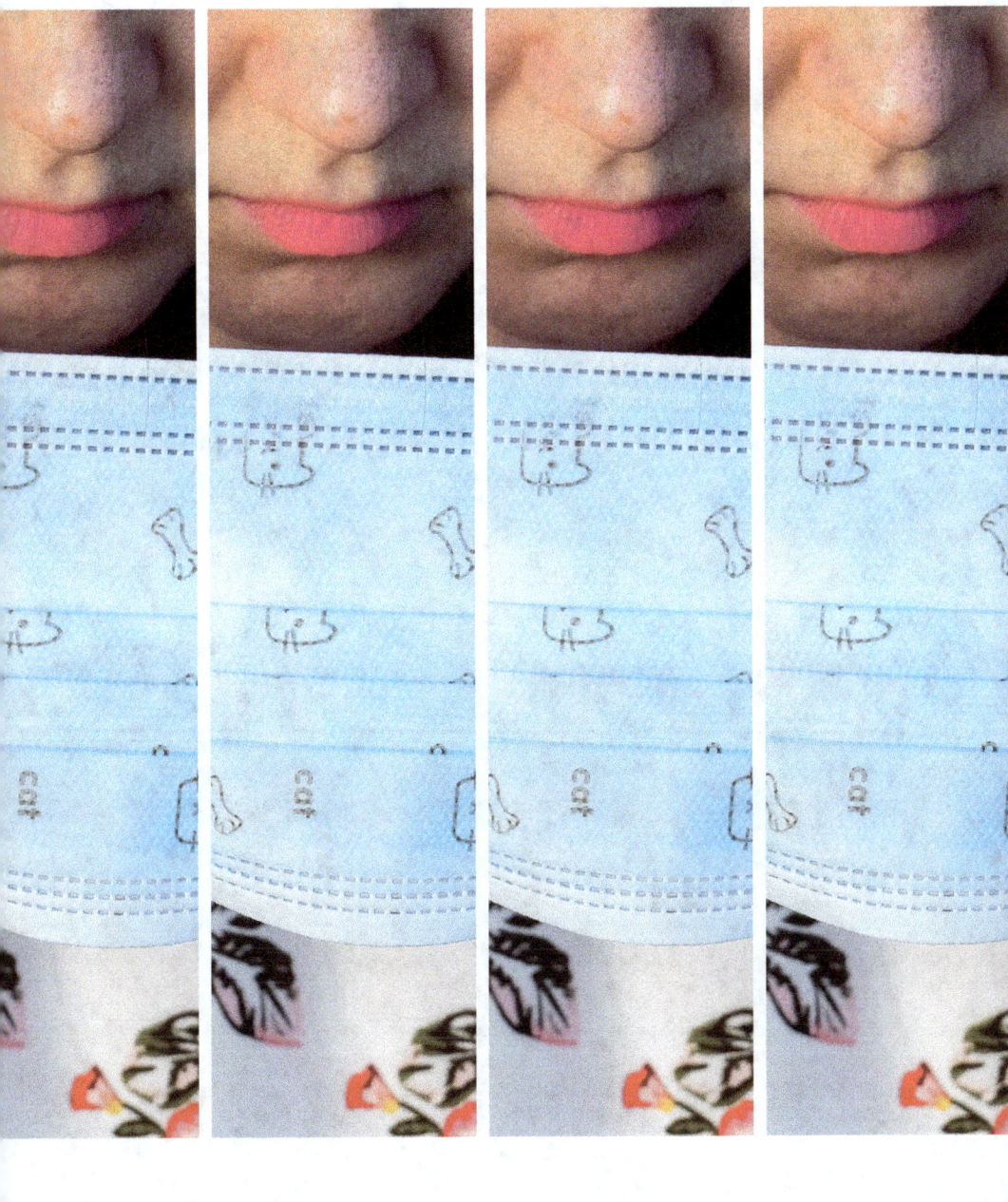

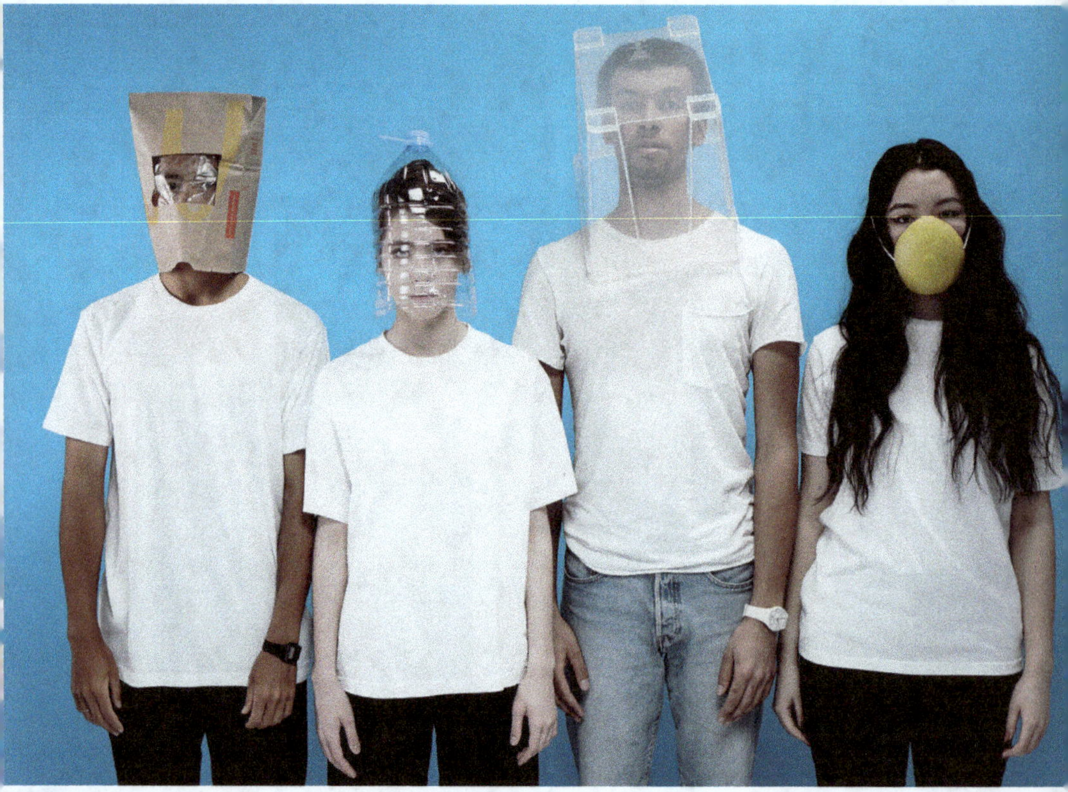

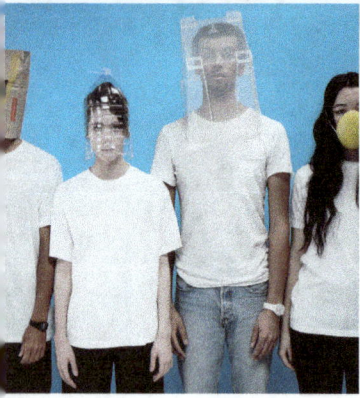
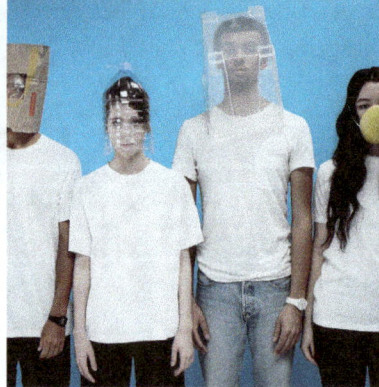
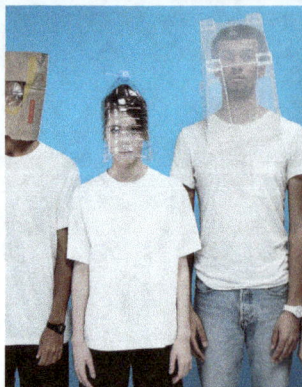

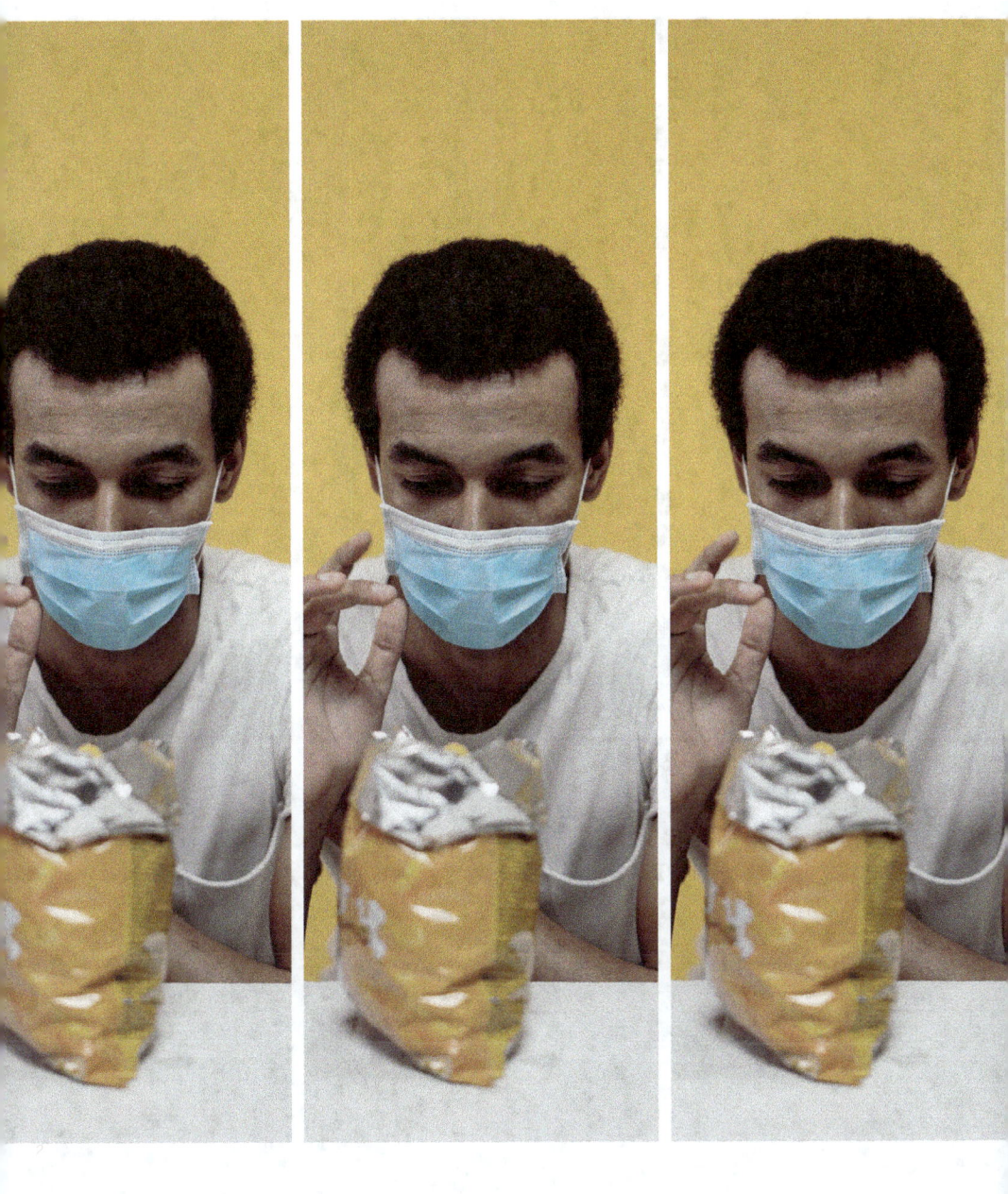

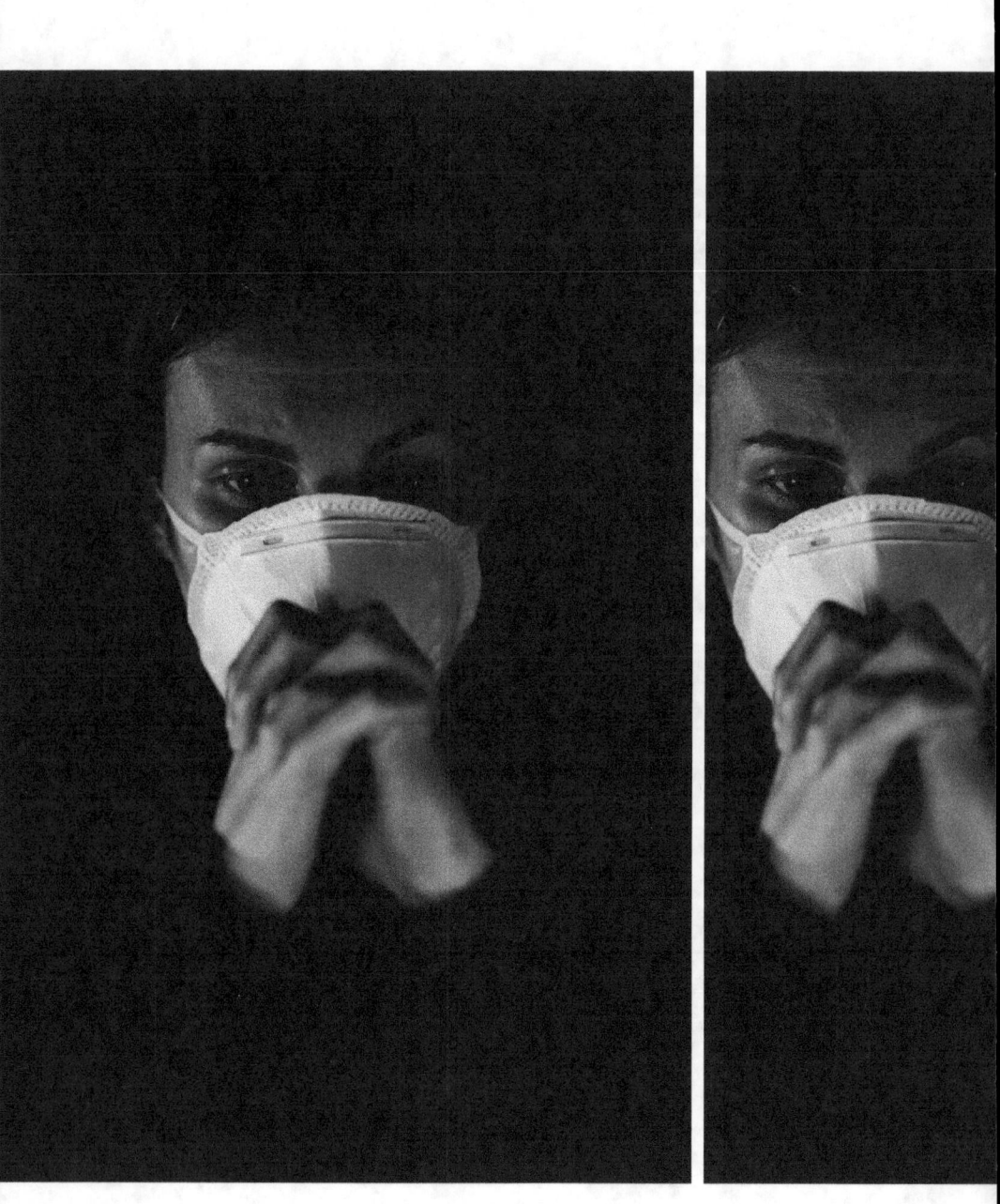

WHEN
IS THE END?
#COVID19

WHEN
IS THE END?
#COVID19

WHEN
IS THE END?
#COVID19

WHEN
IS THE END?
#COVID19

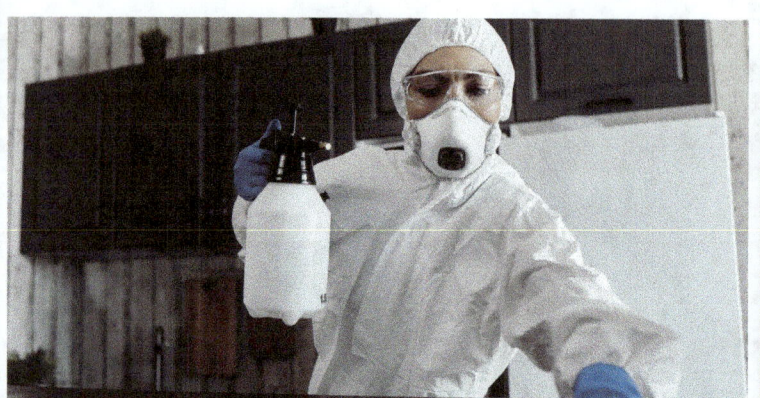
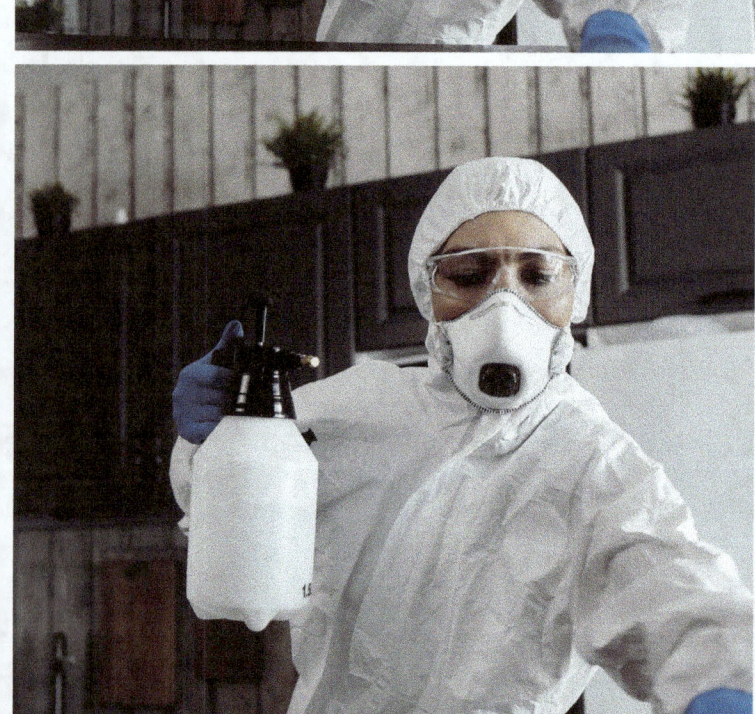
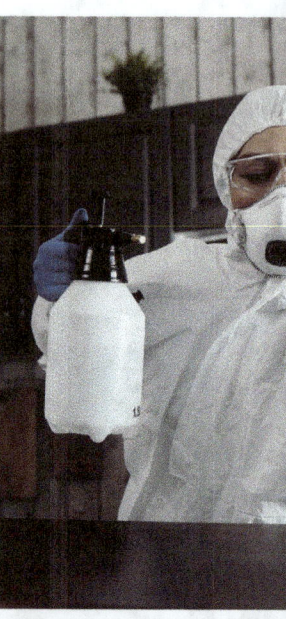
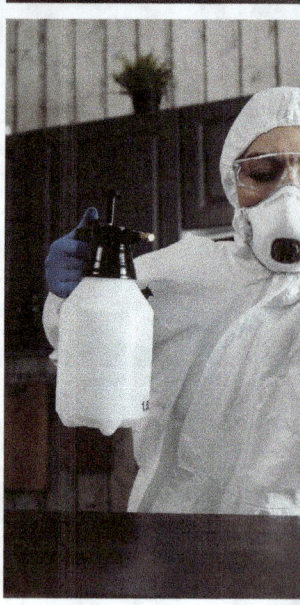

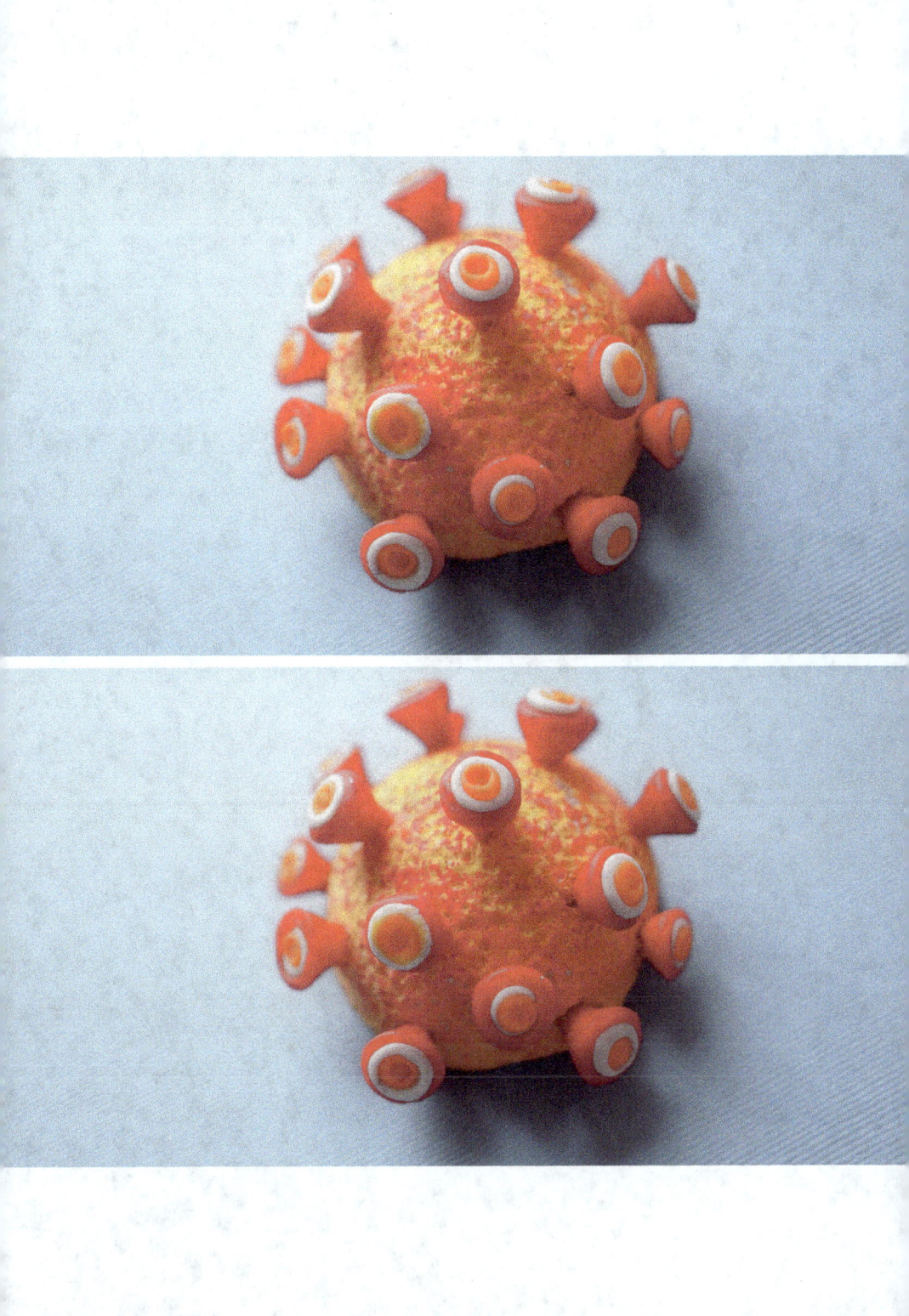

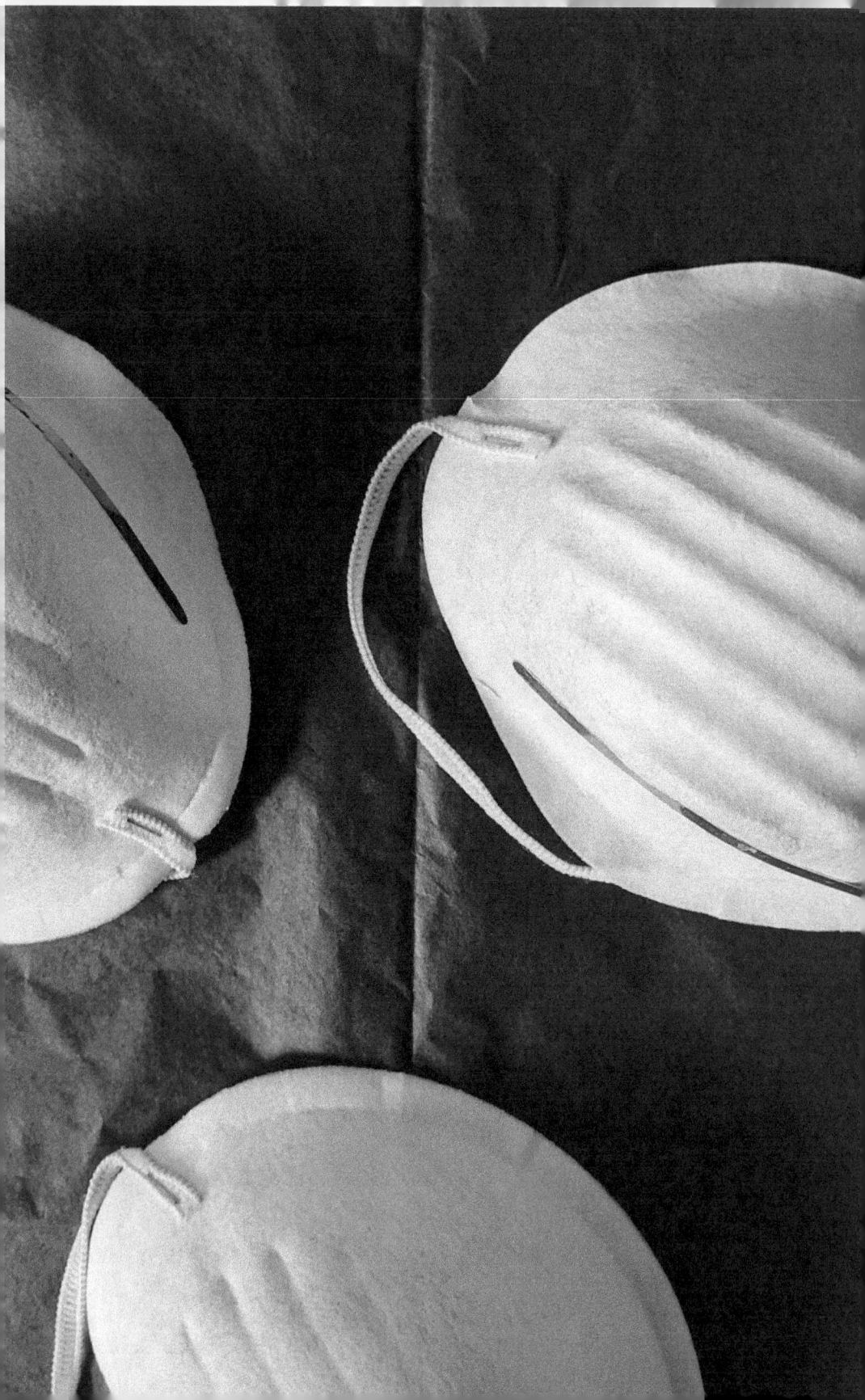

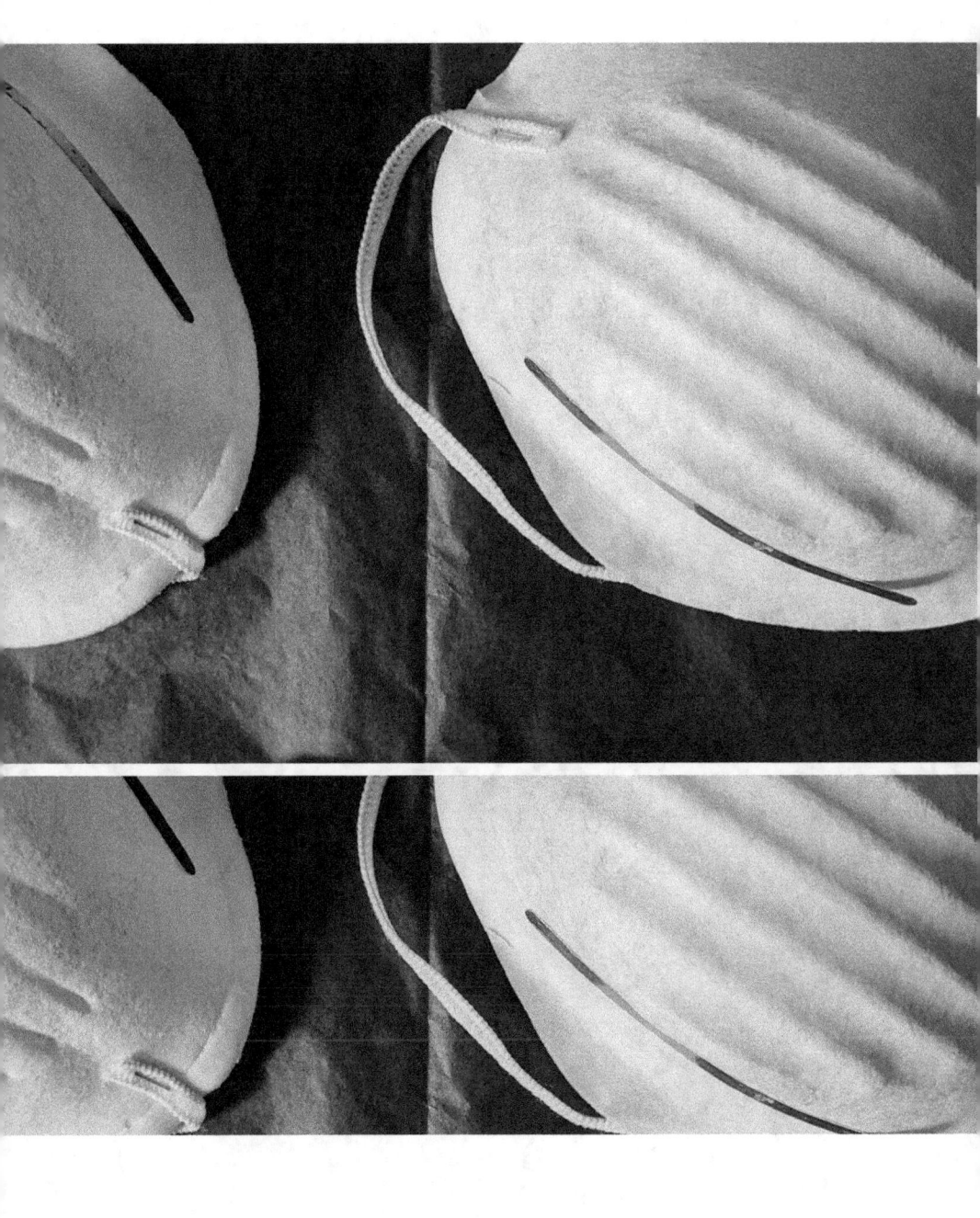

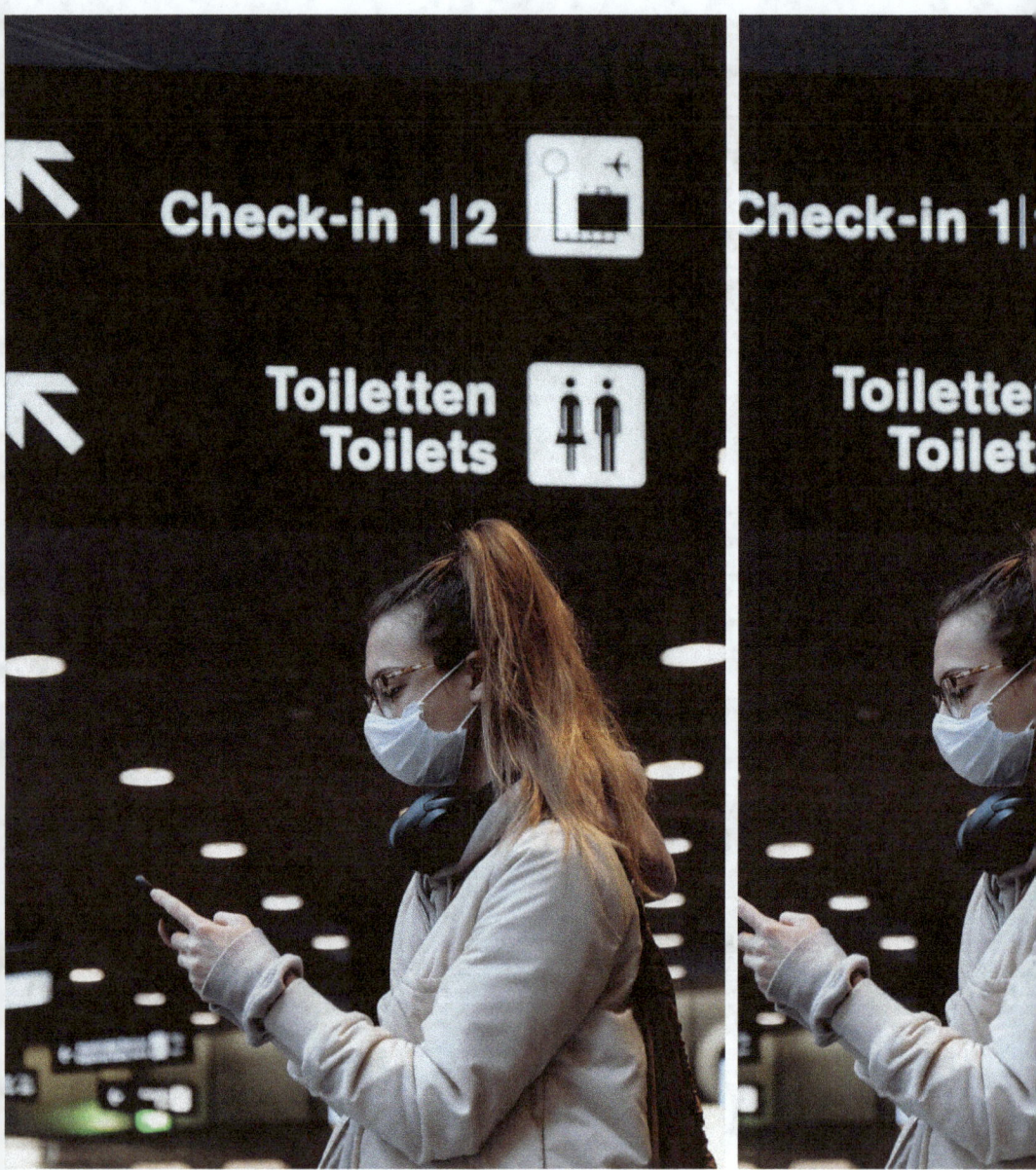

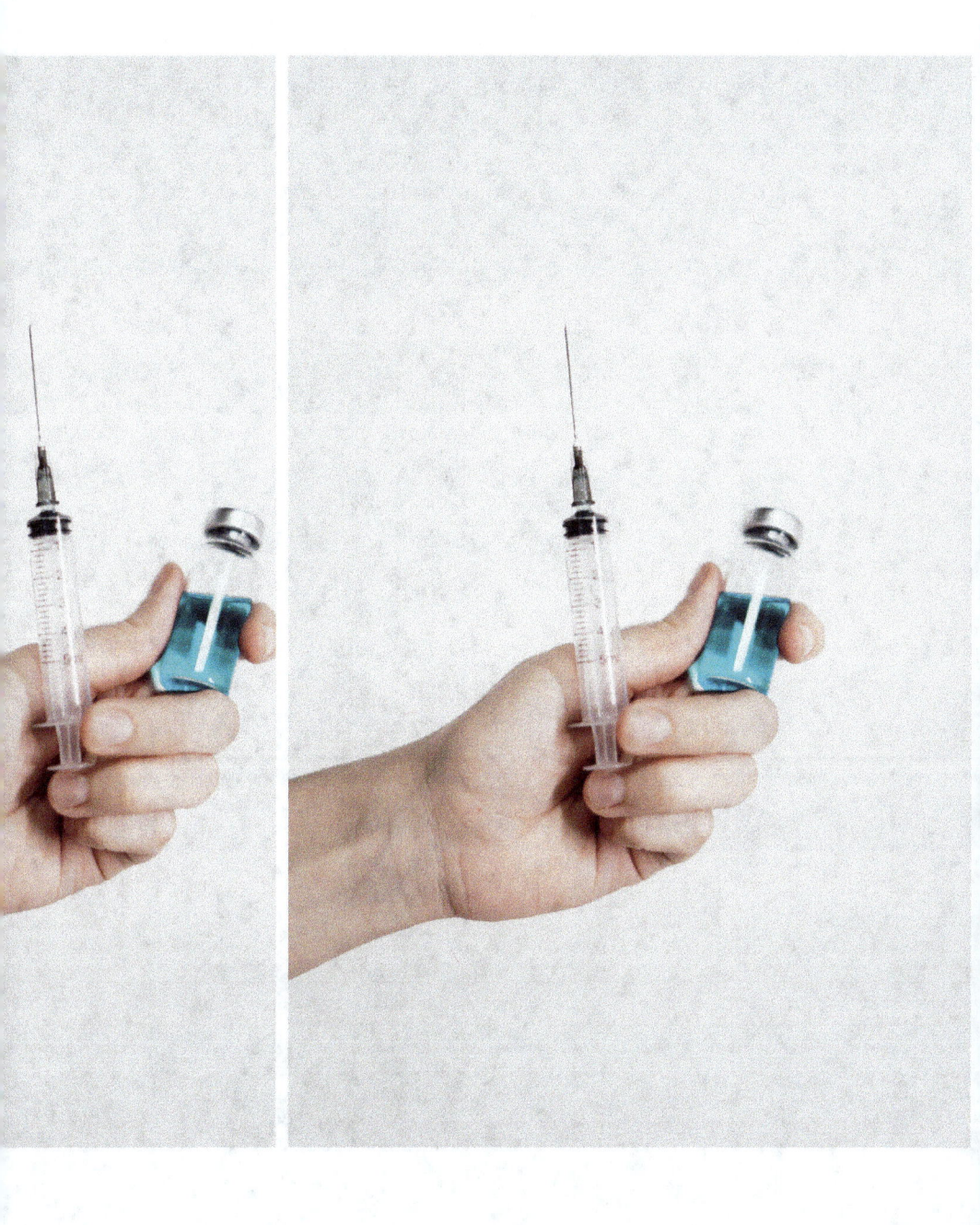

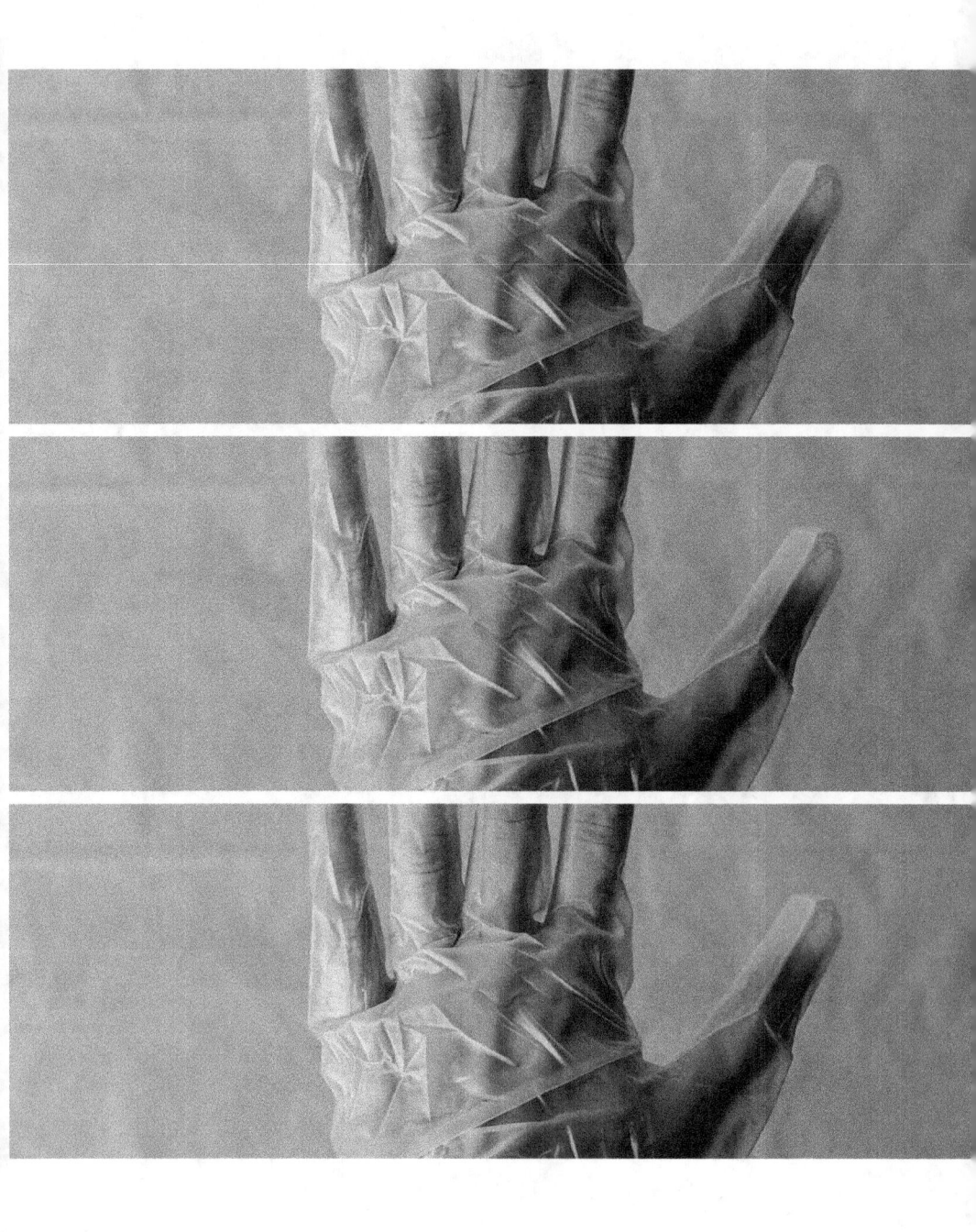

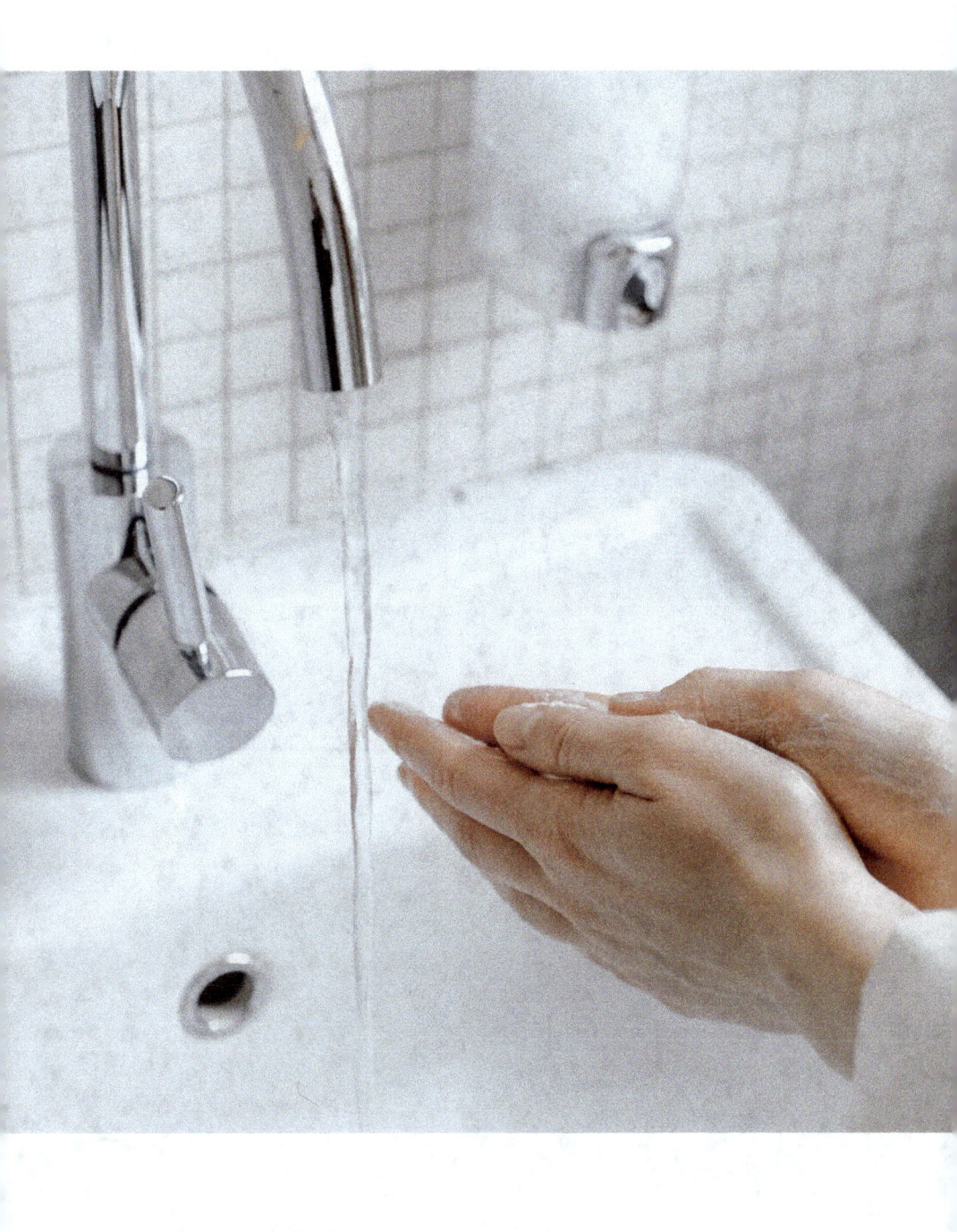

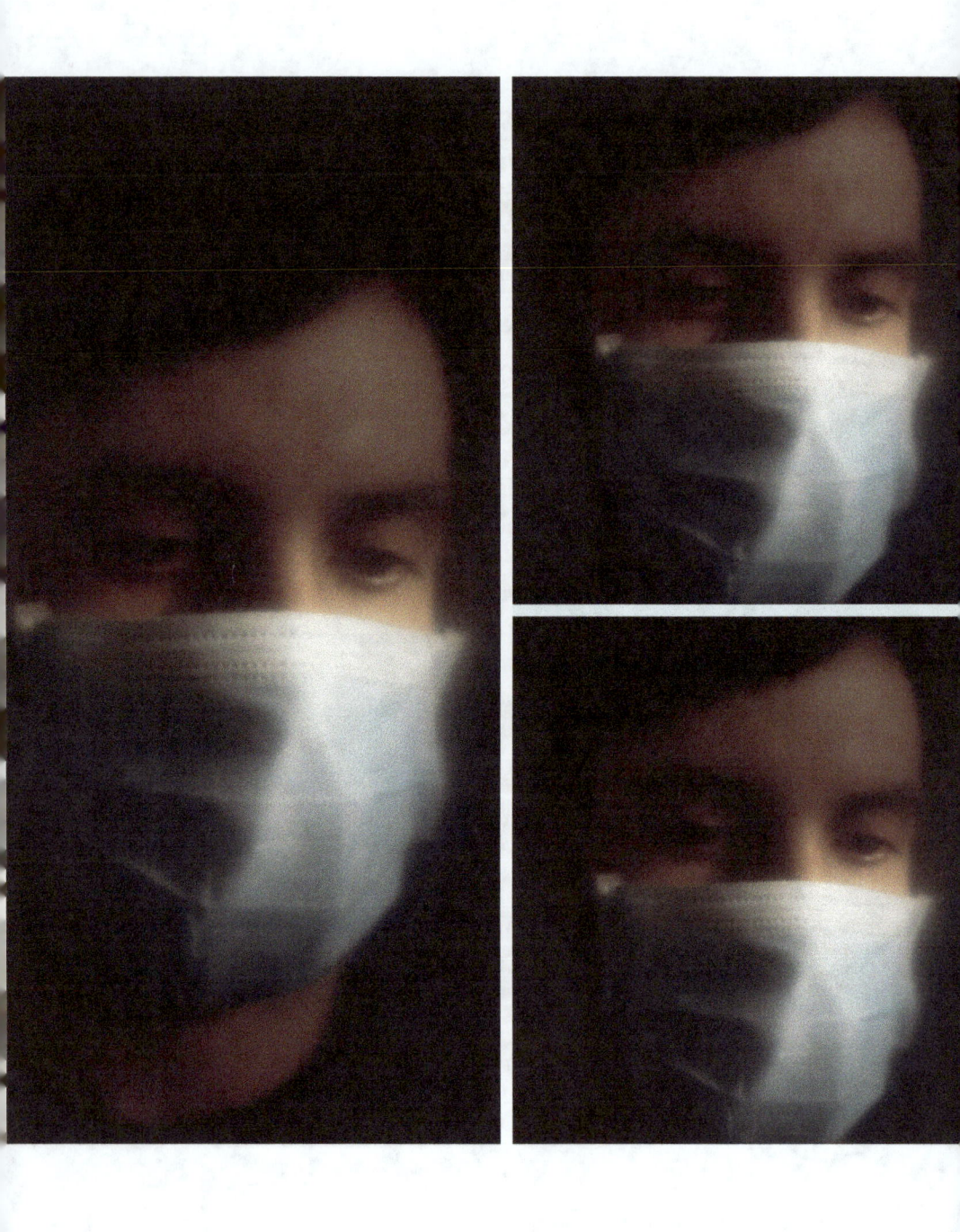

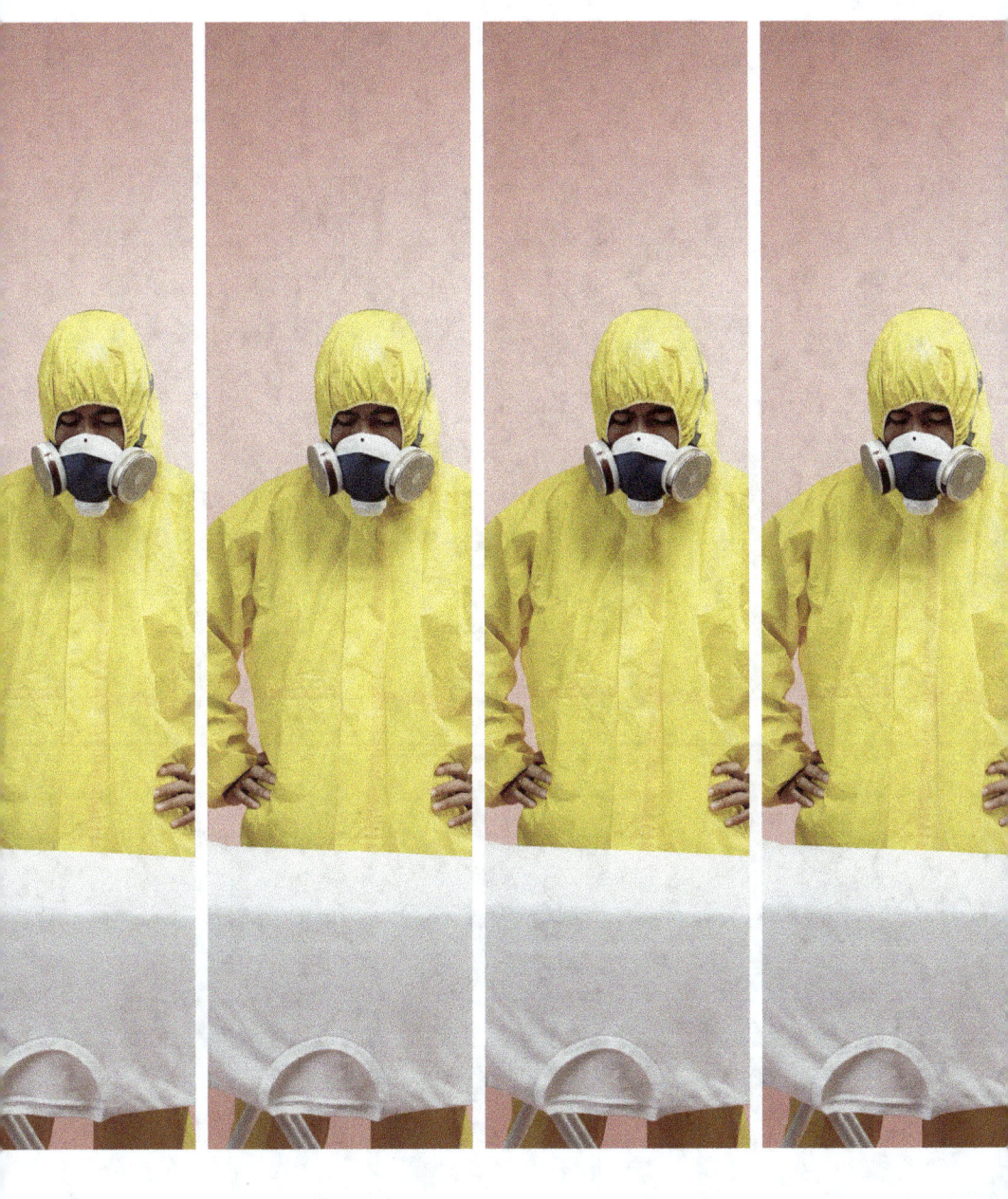

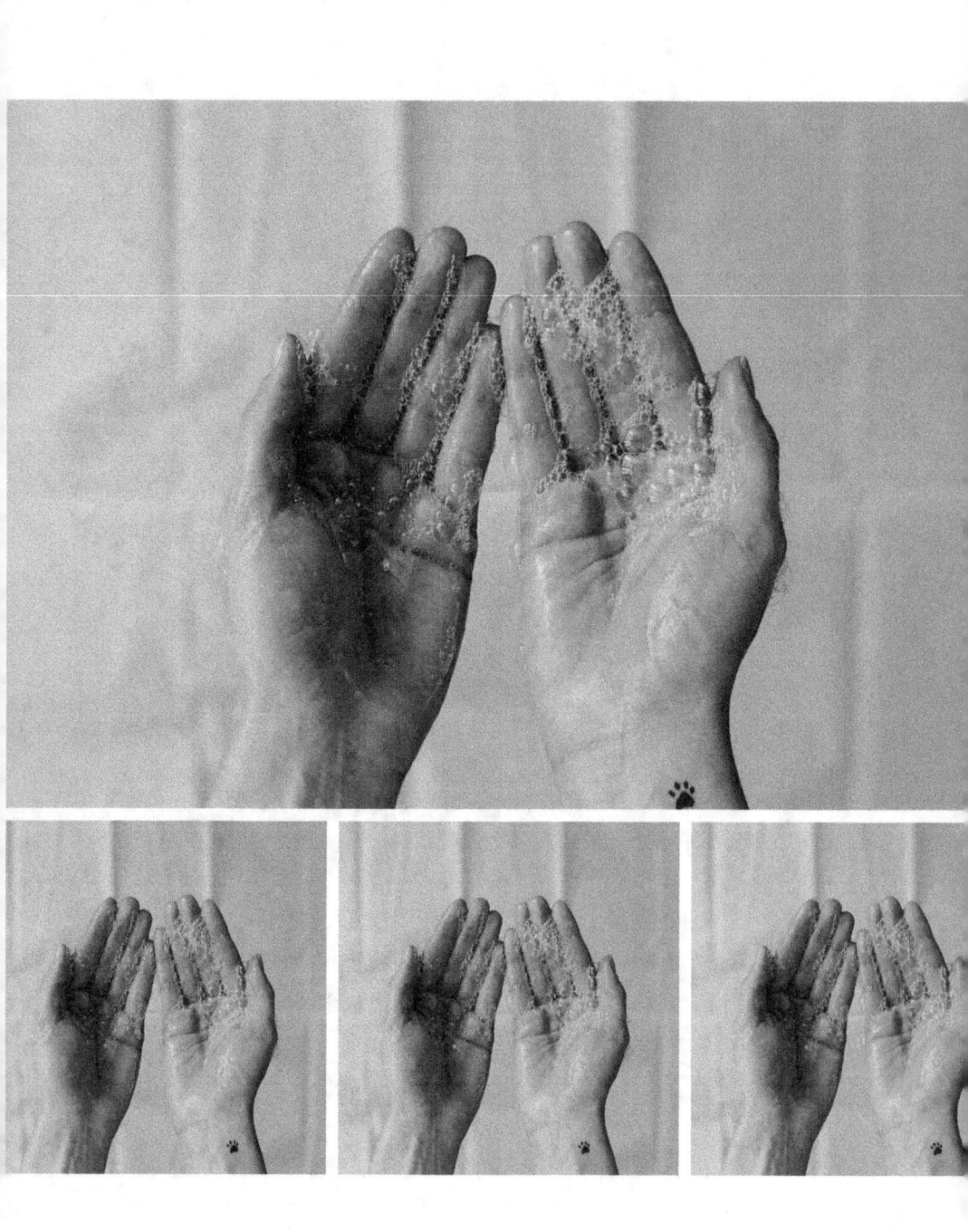

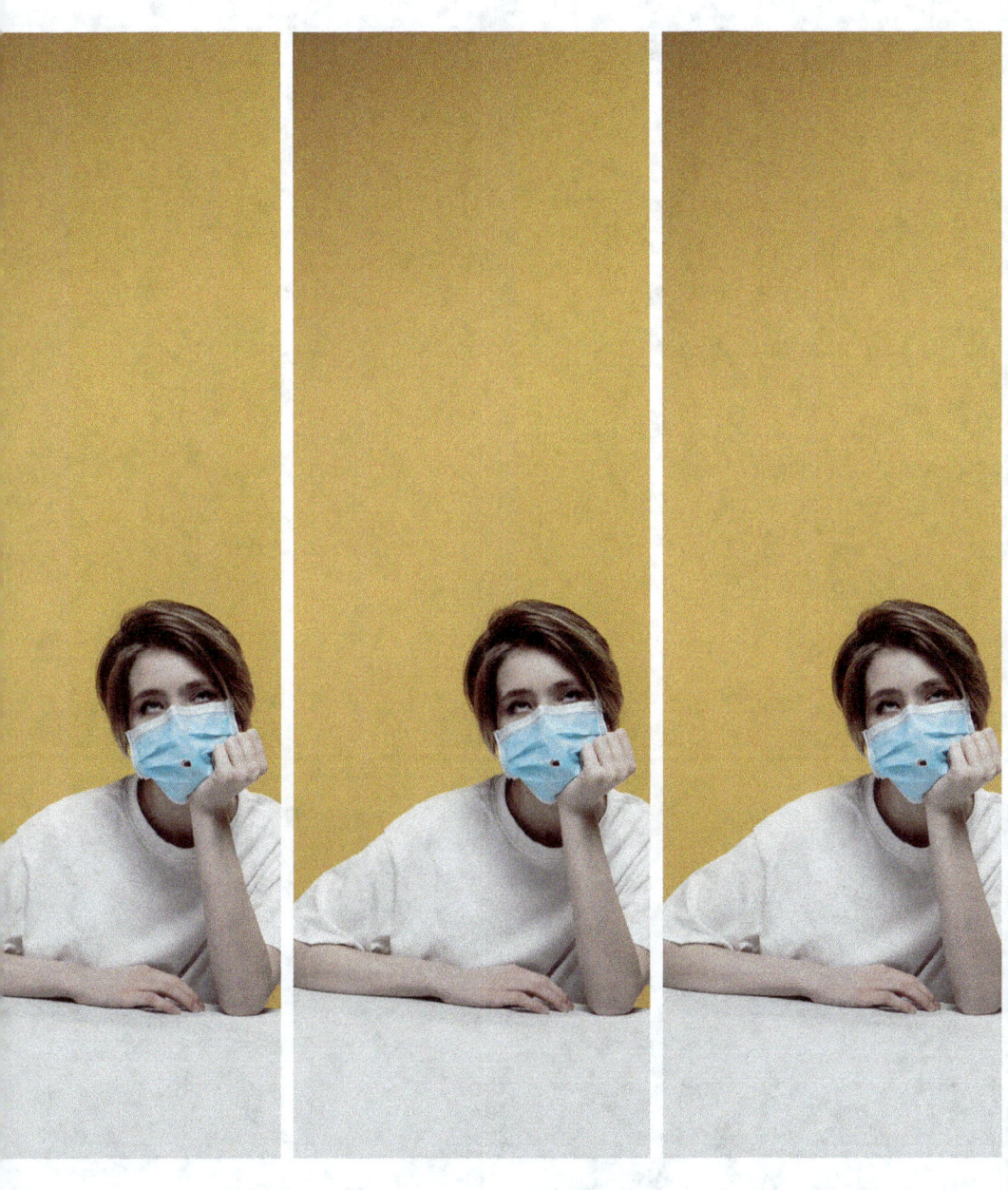

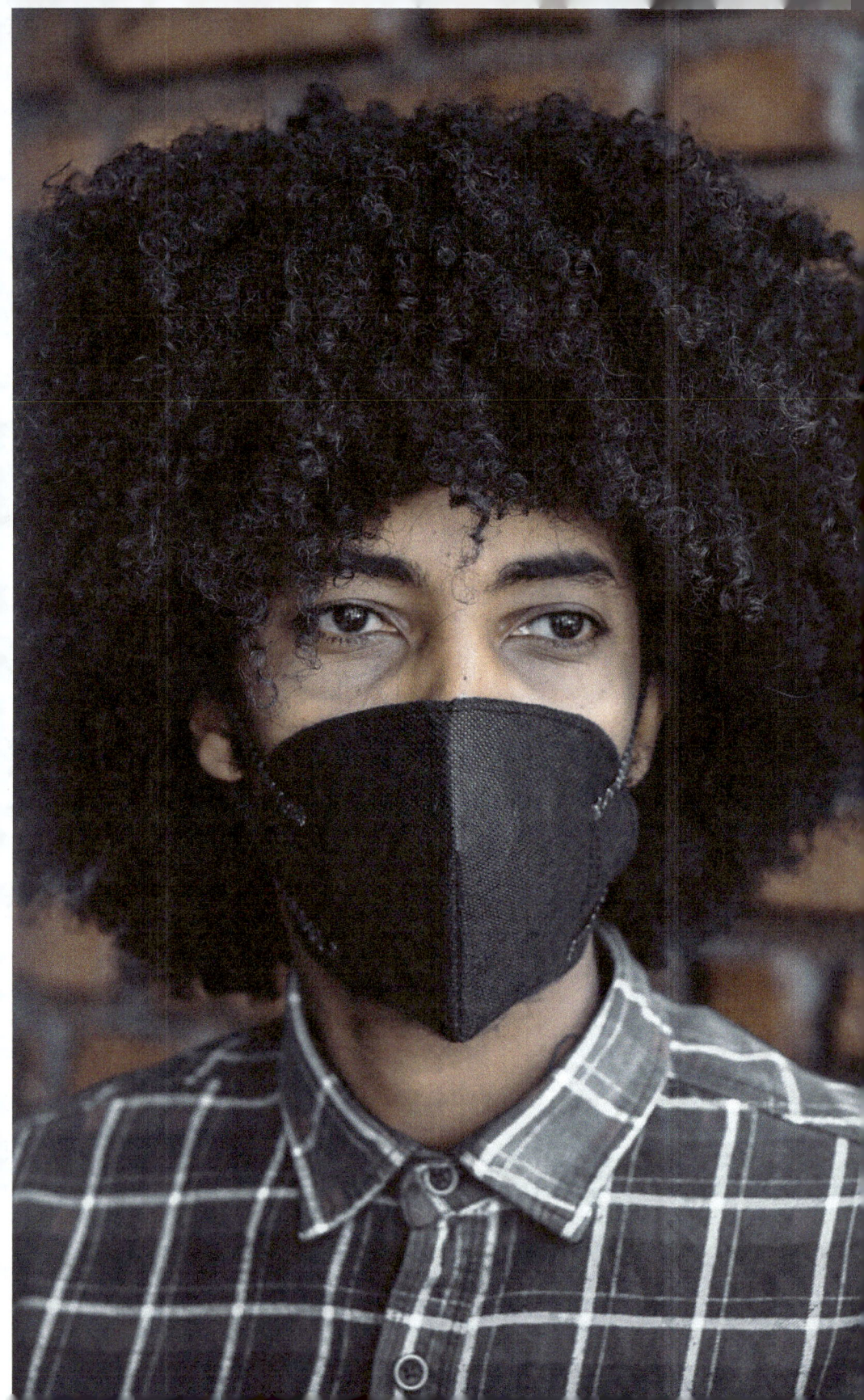

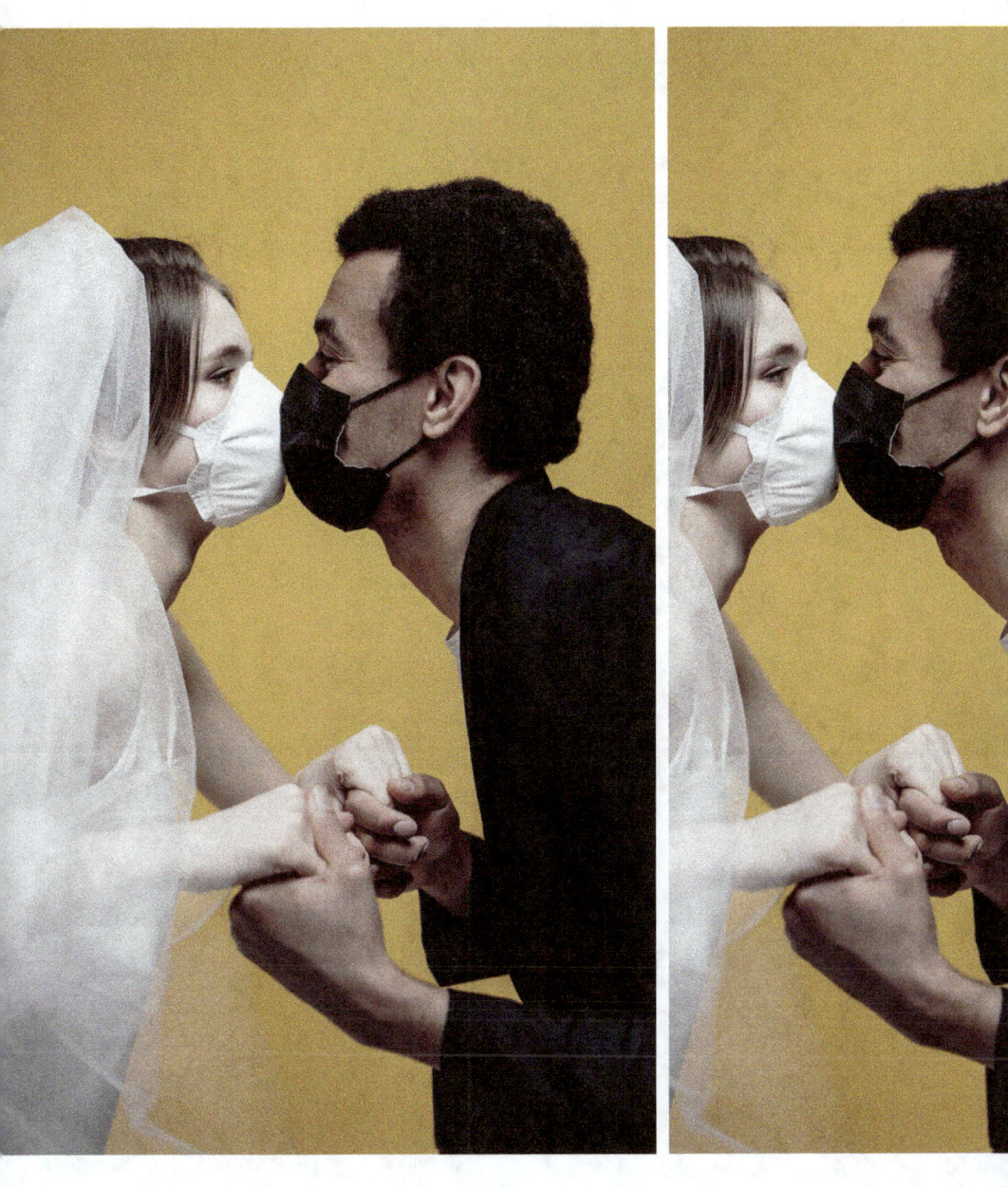

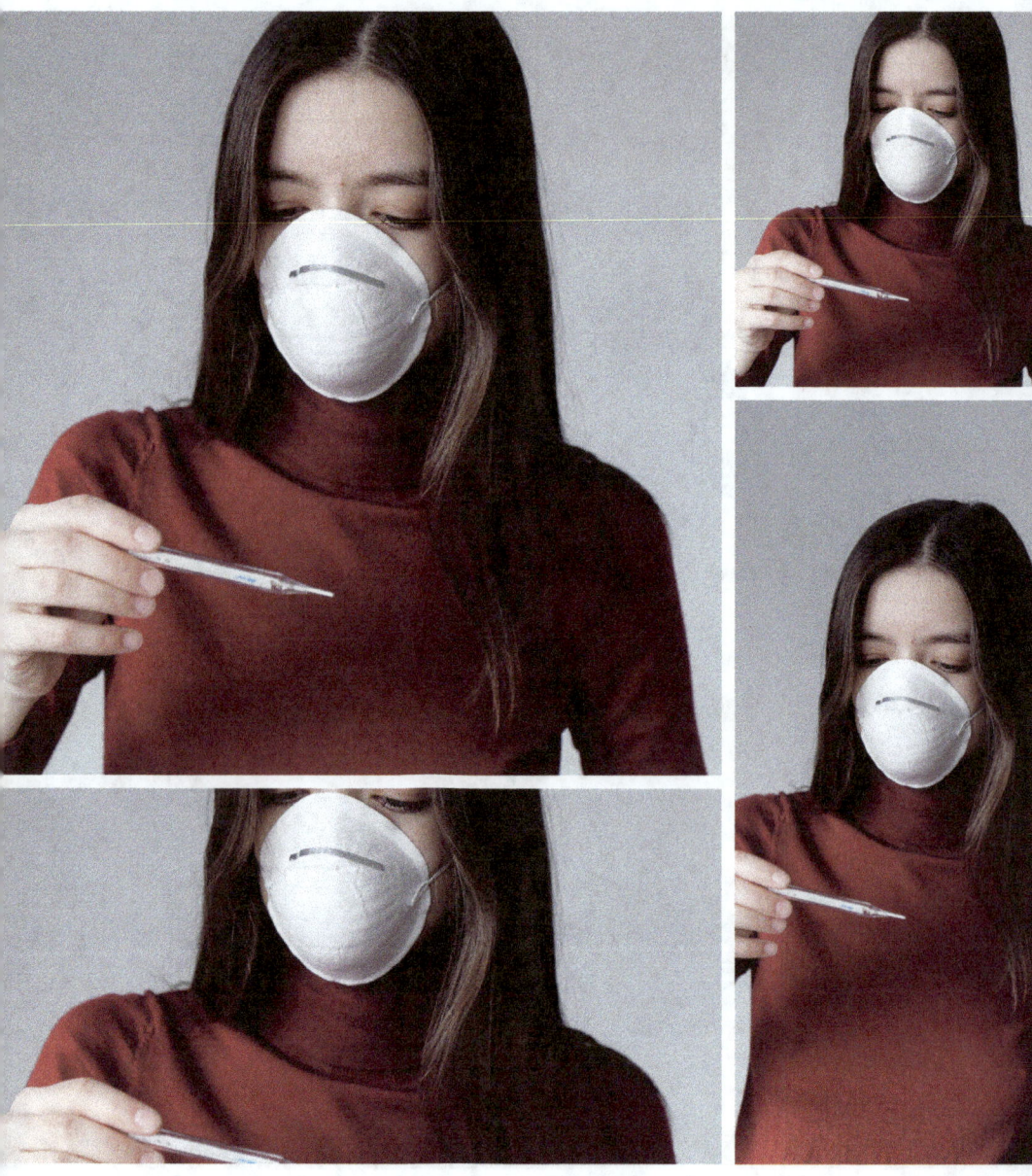

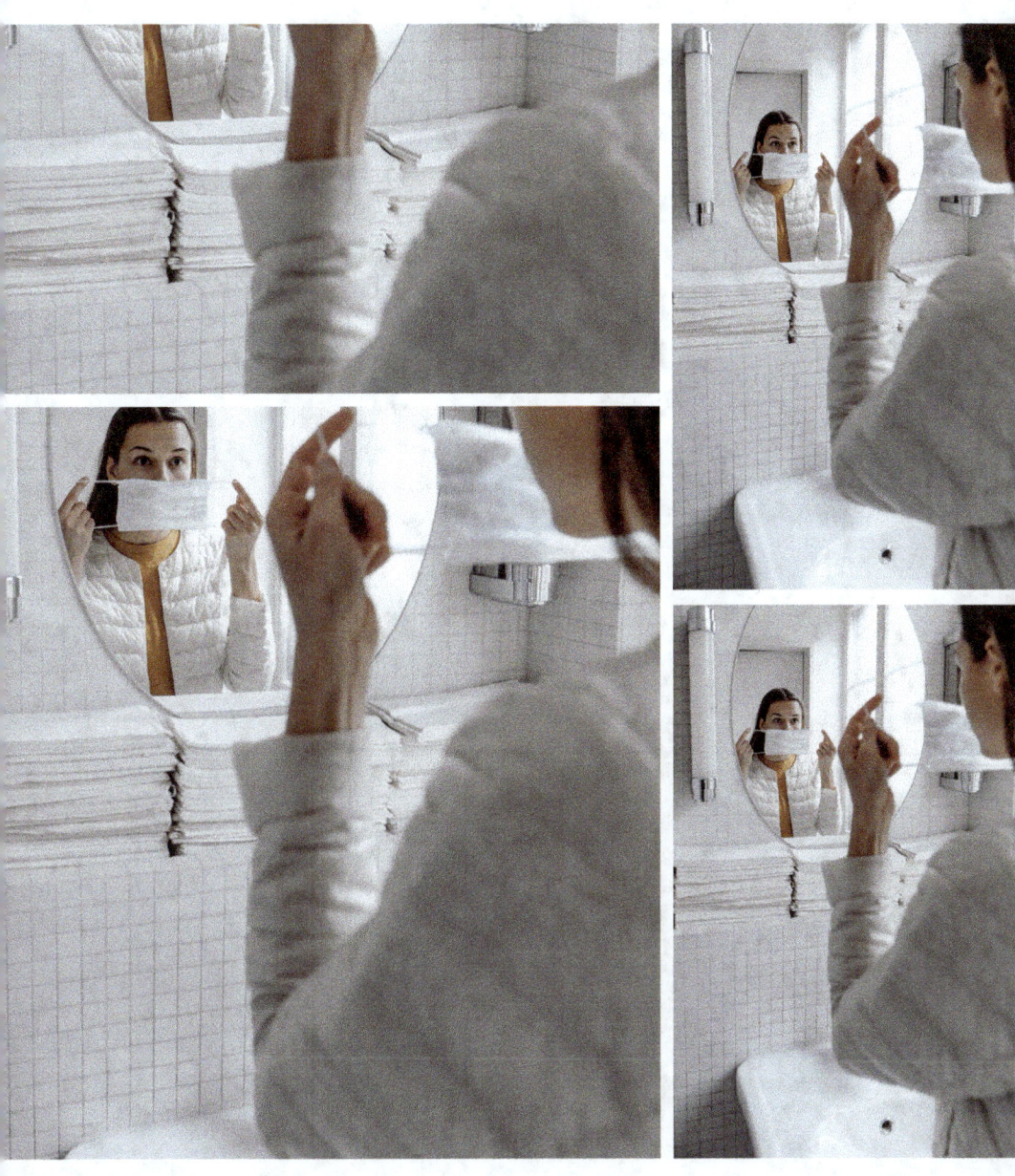

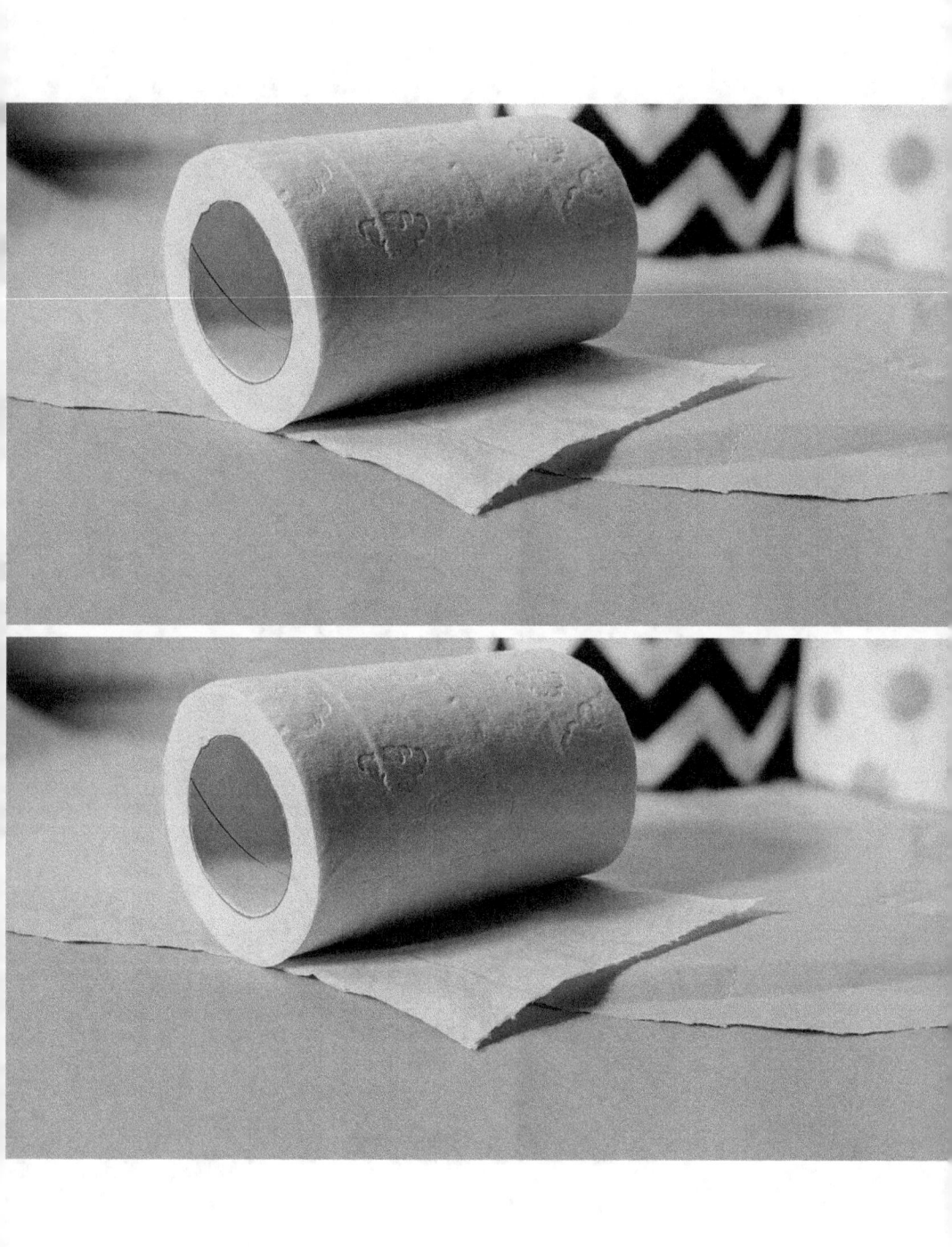

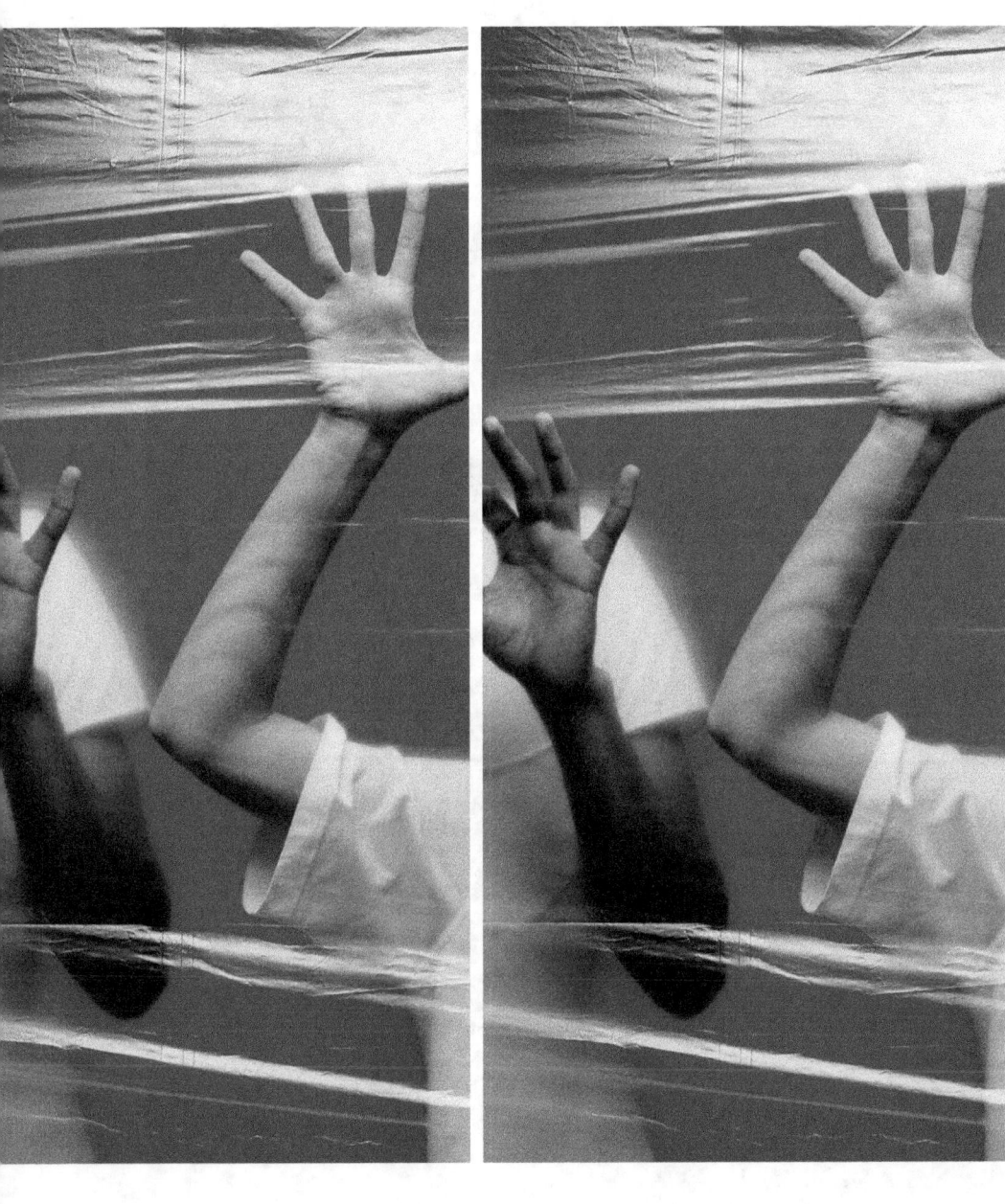

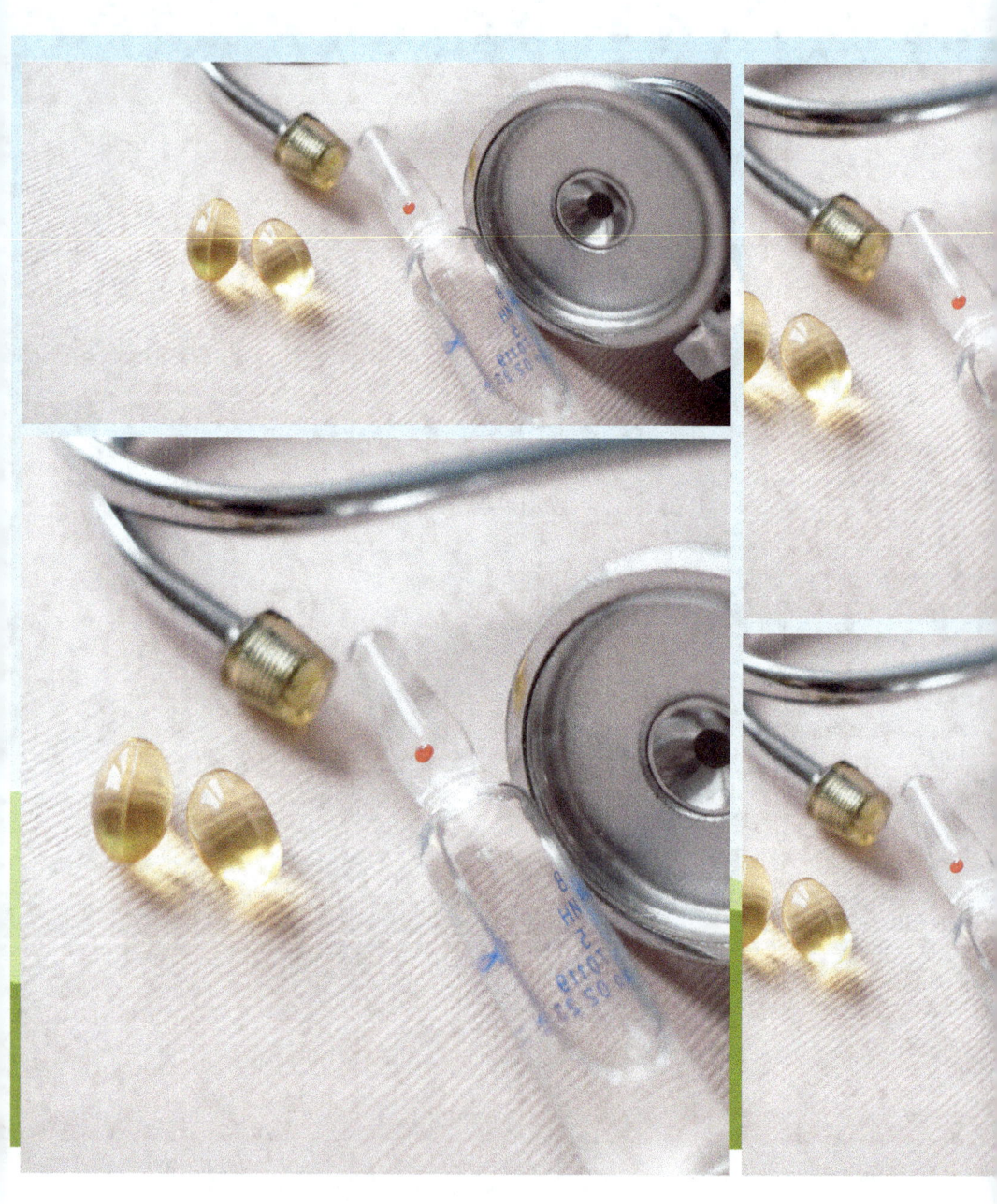

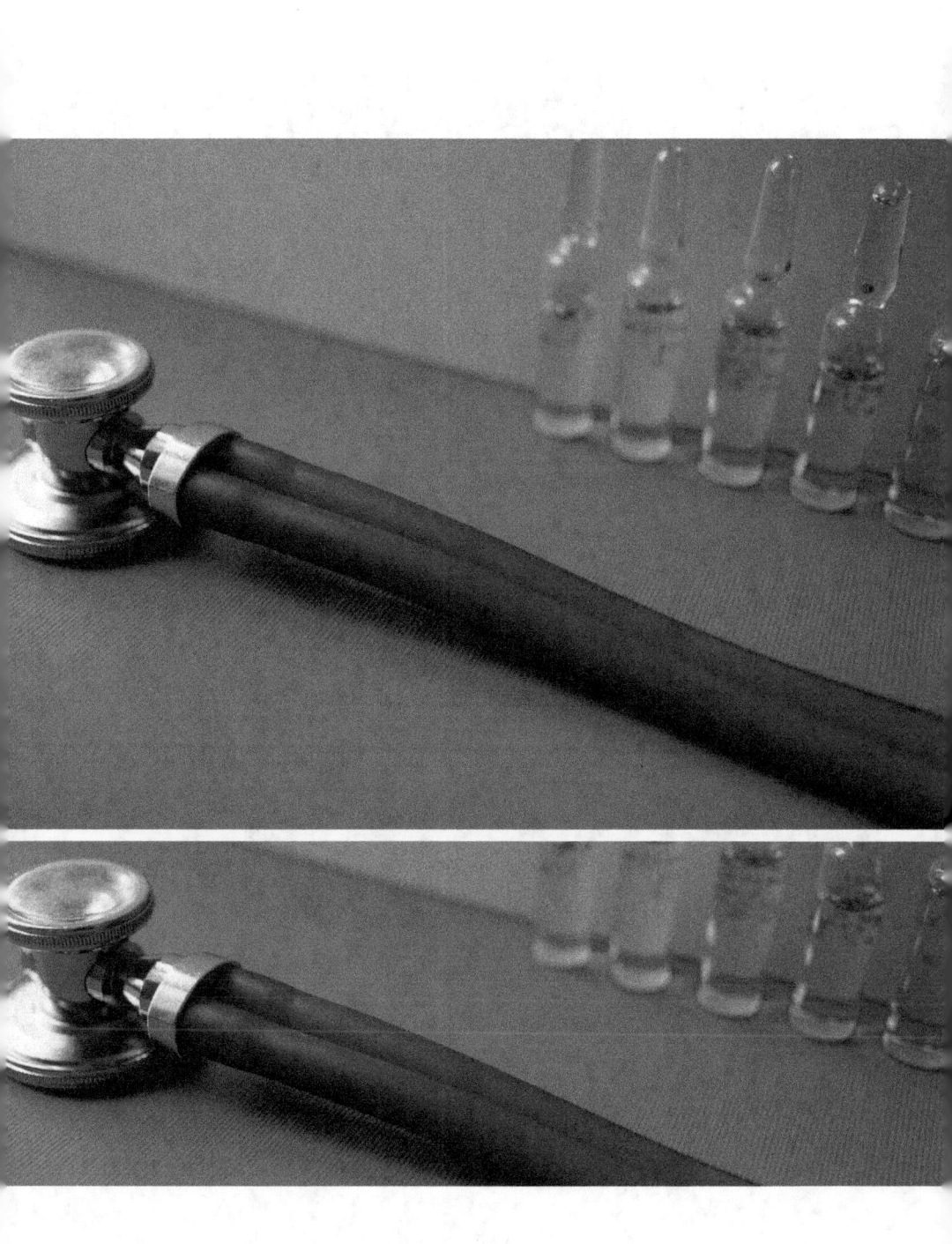

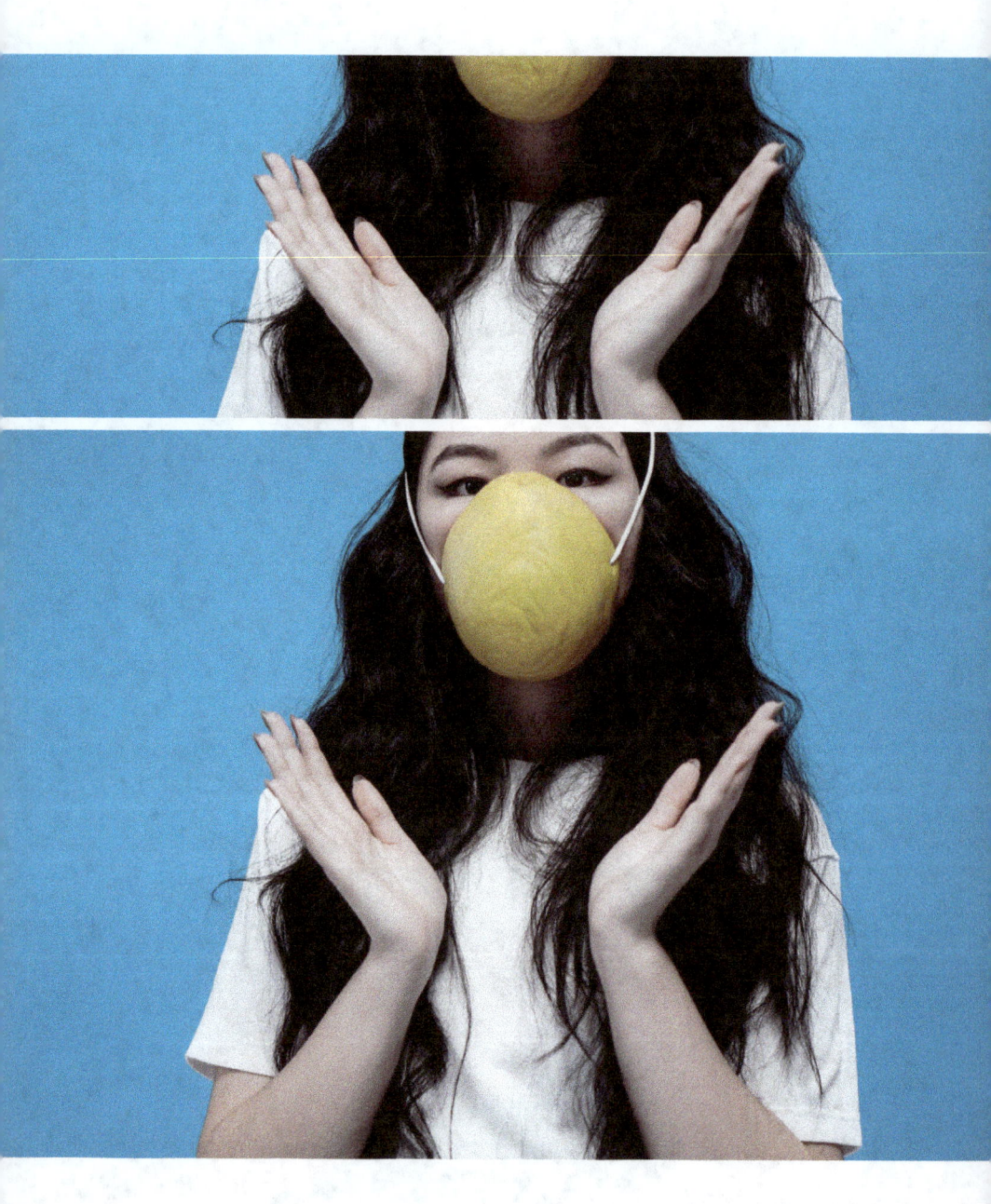

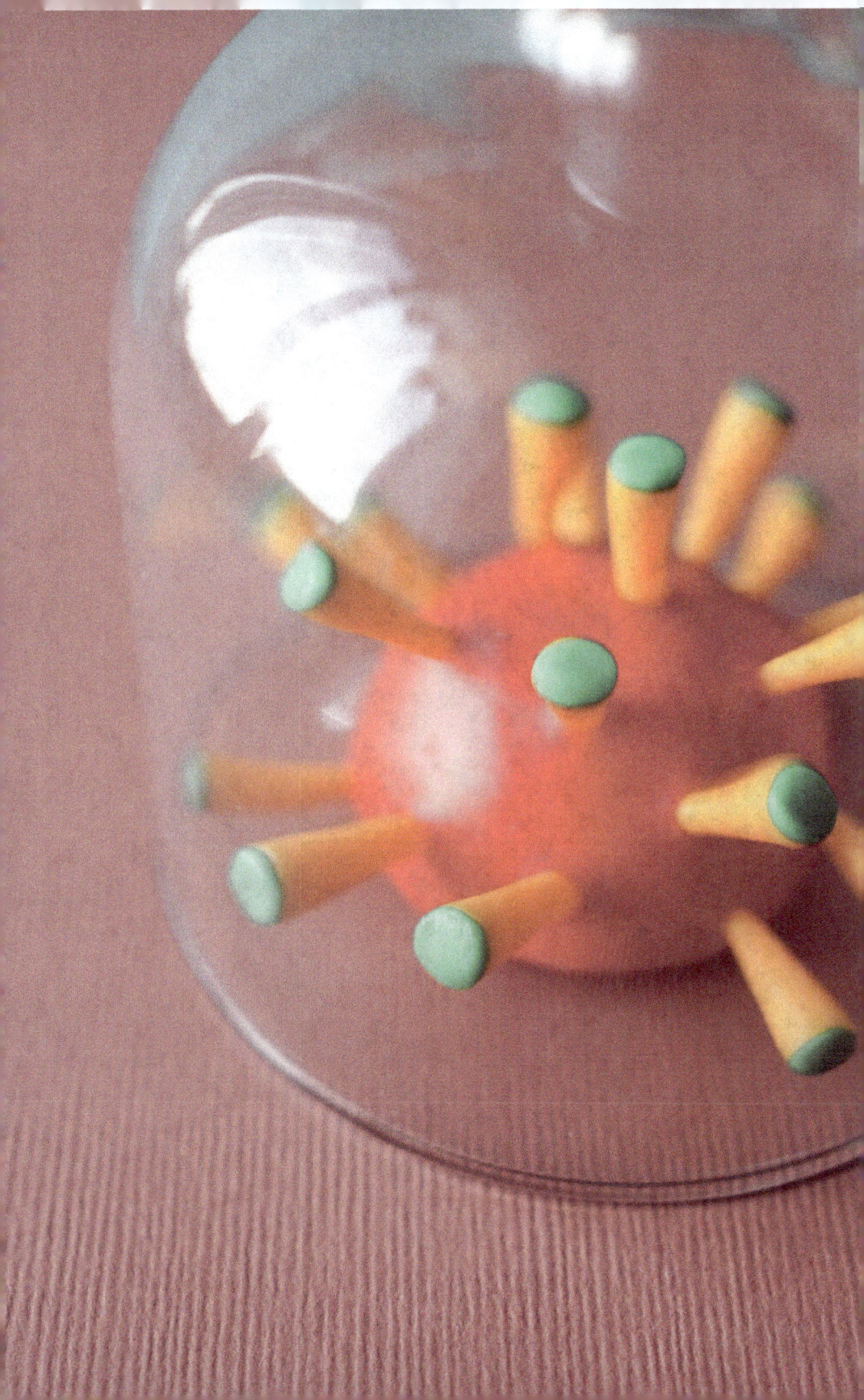

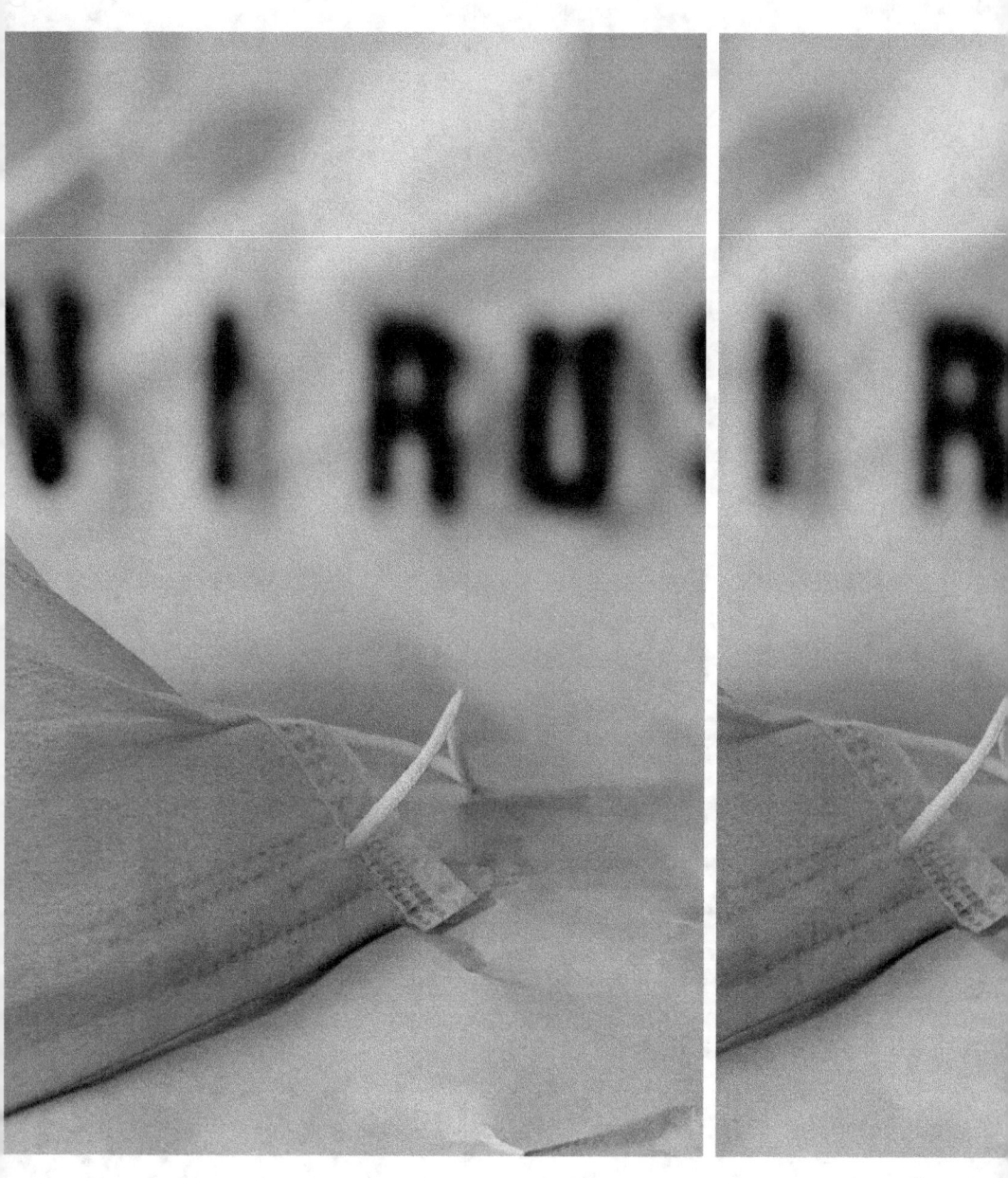

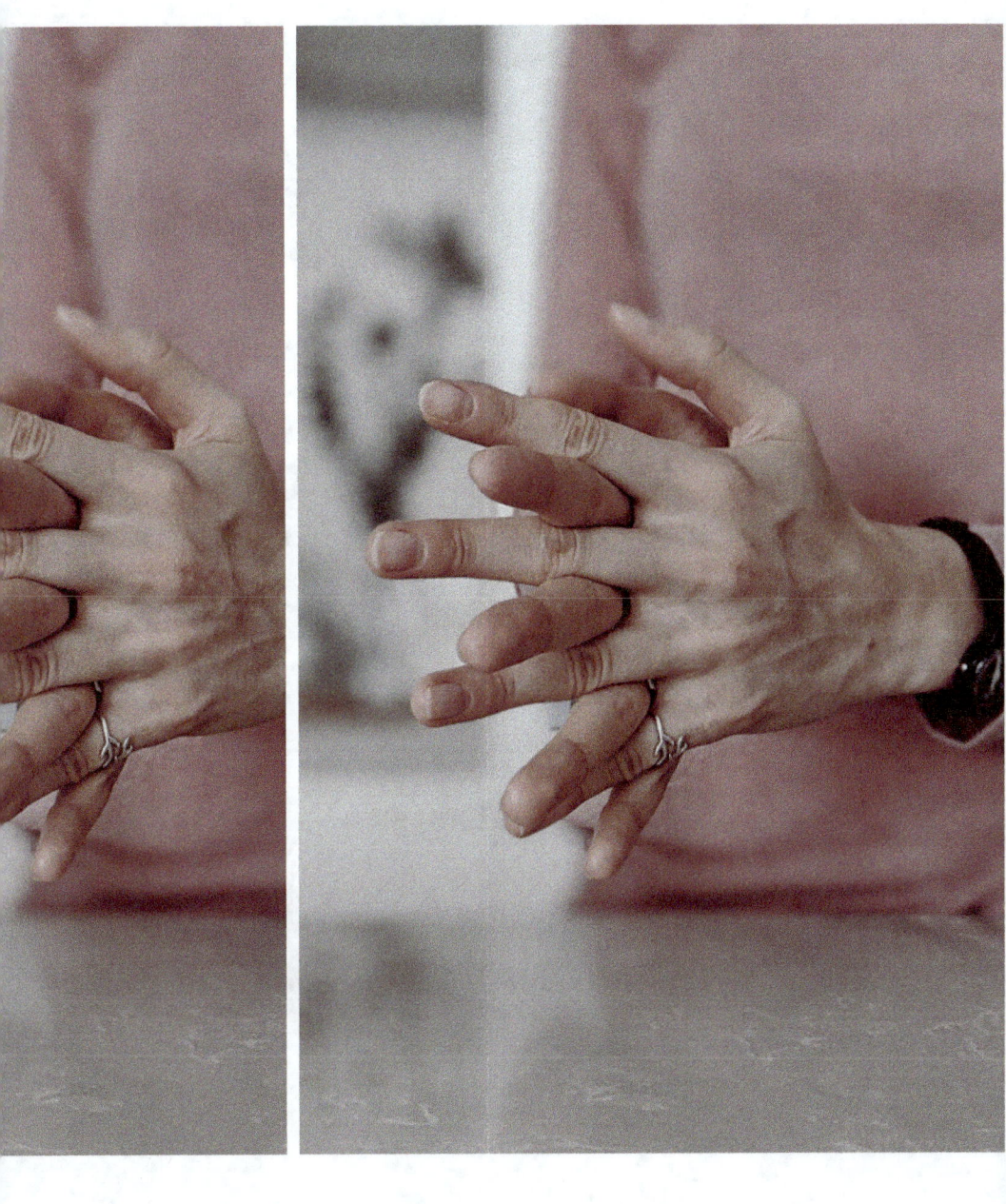

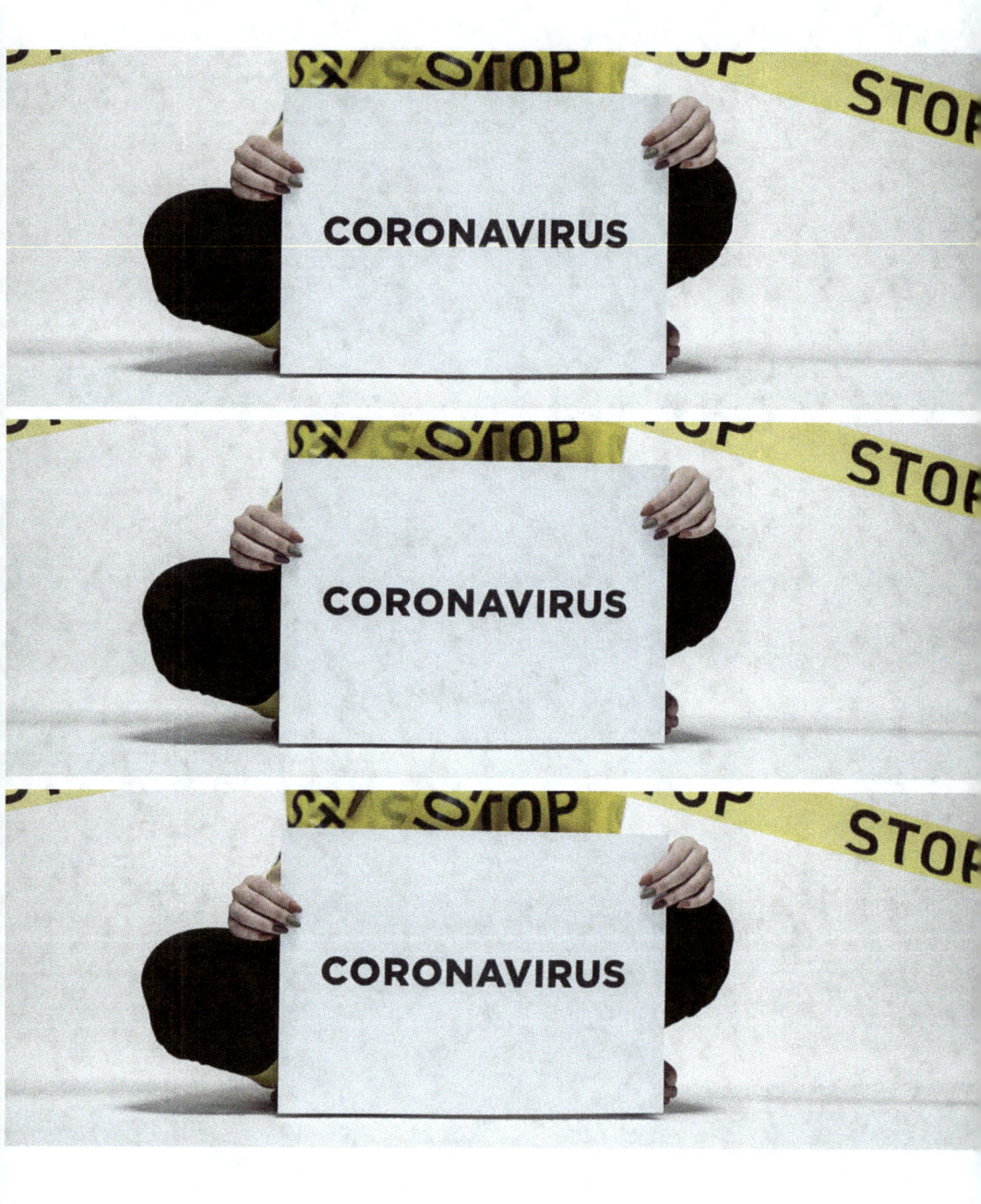

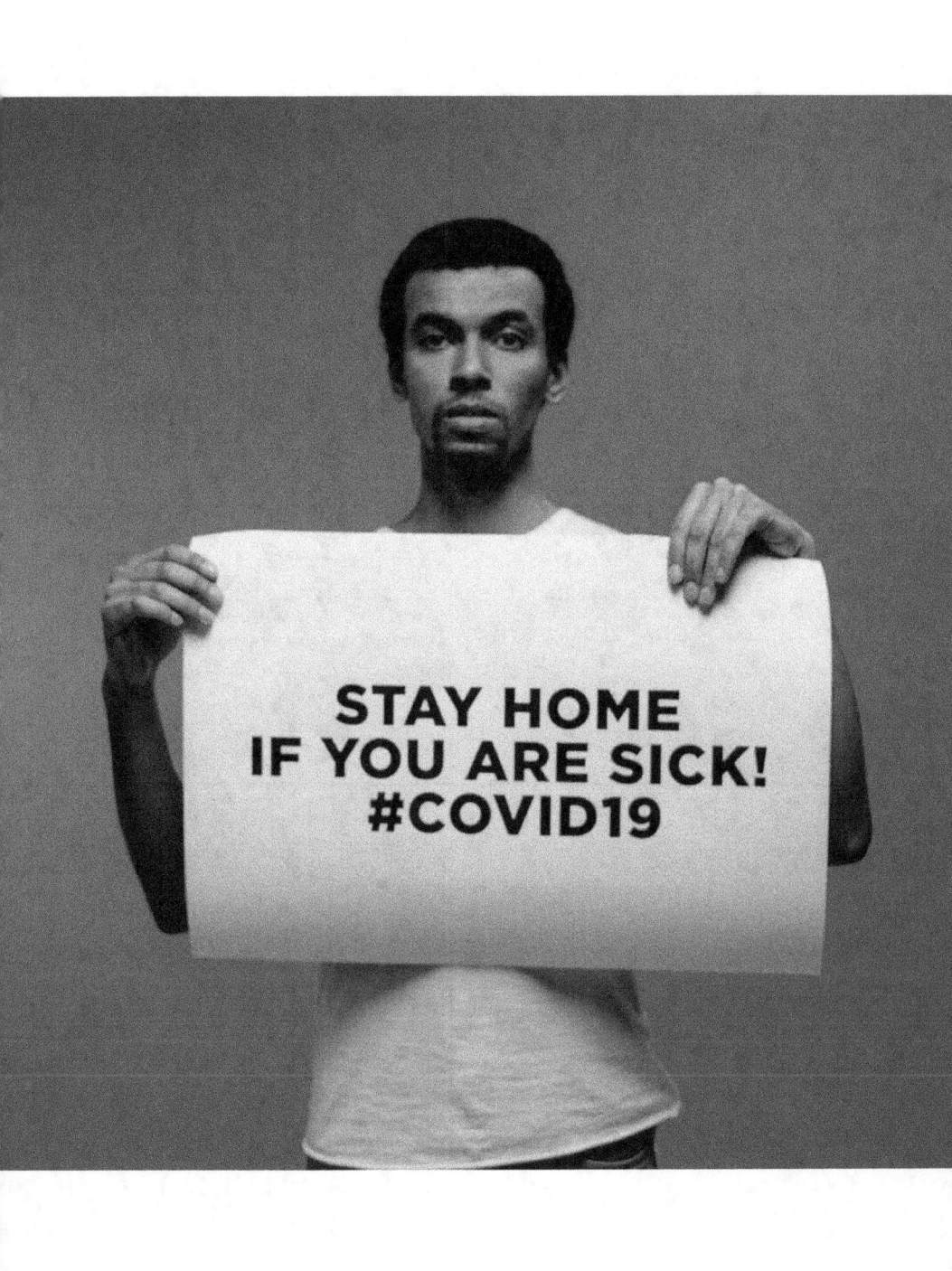

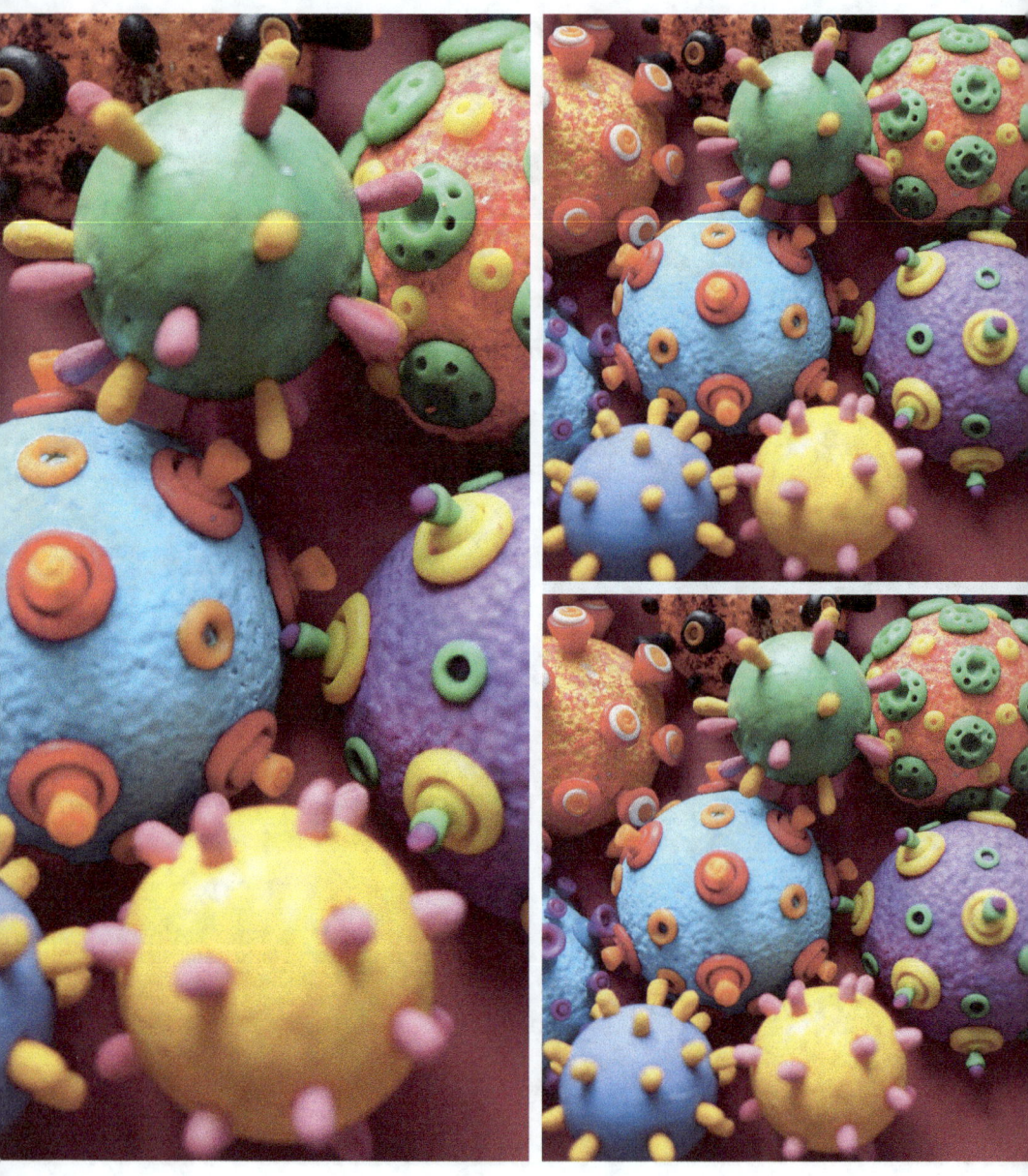

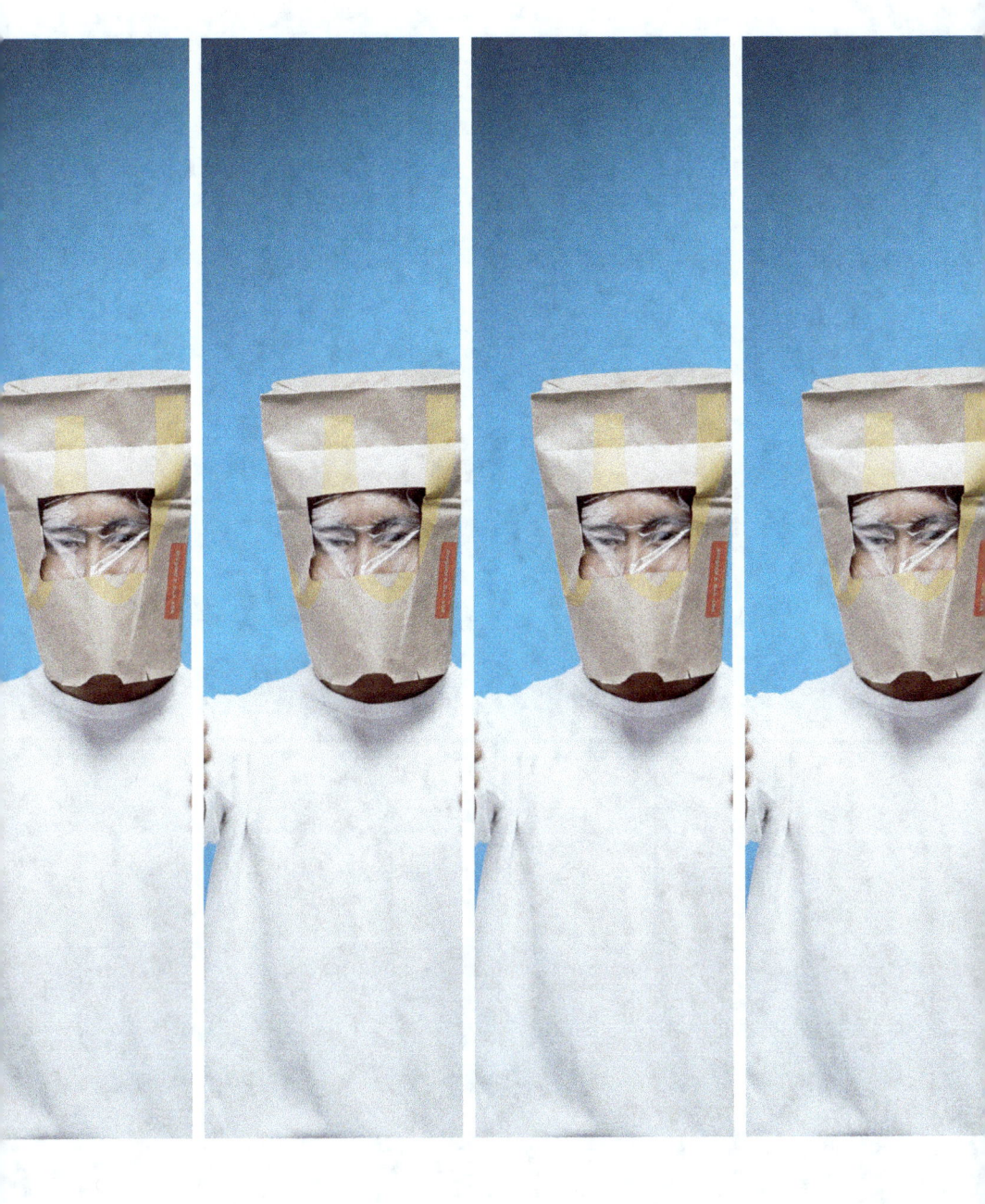

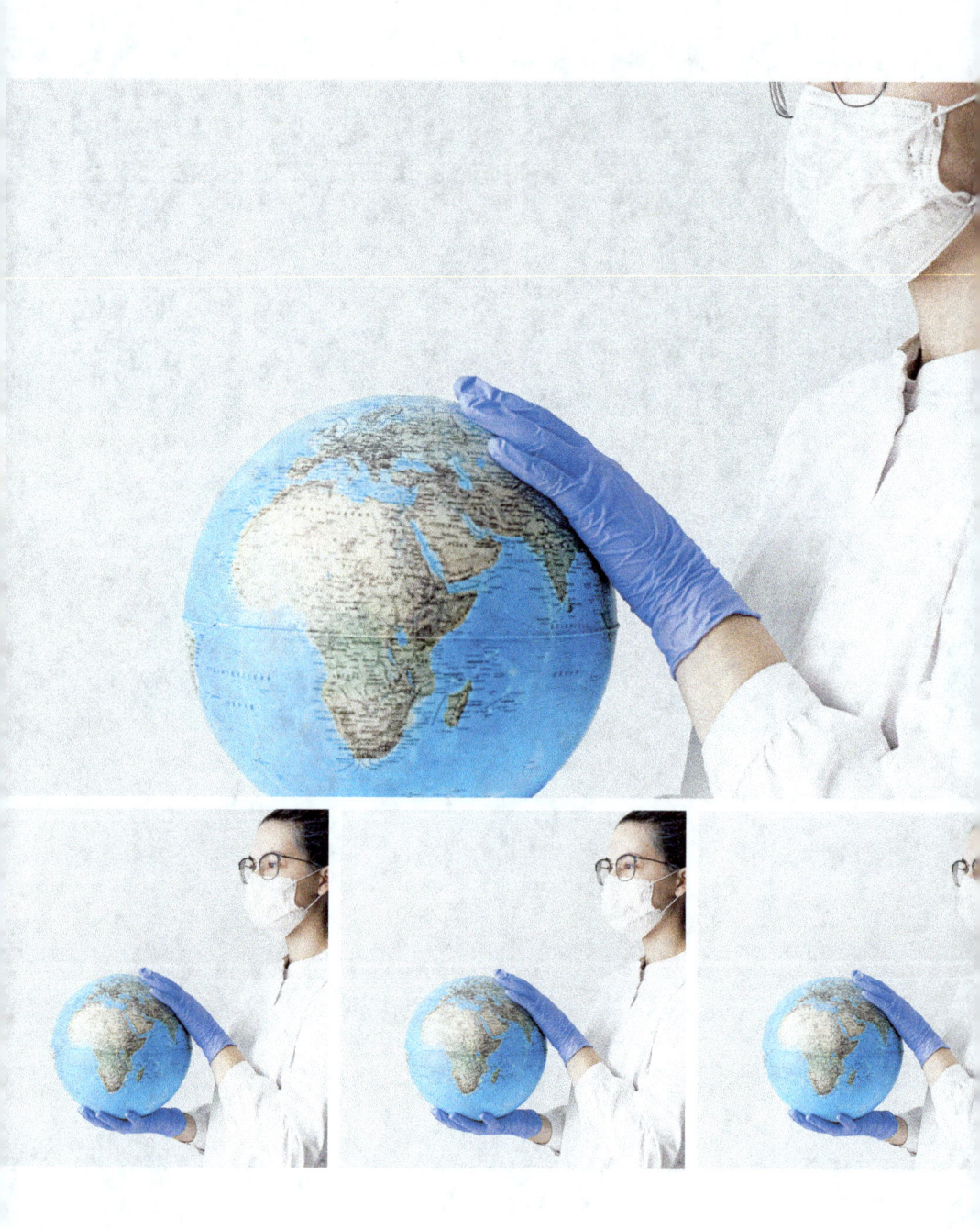

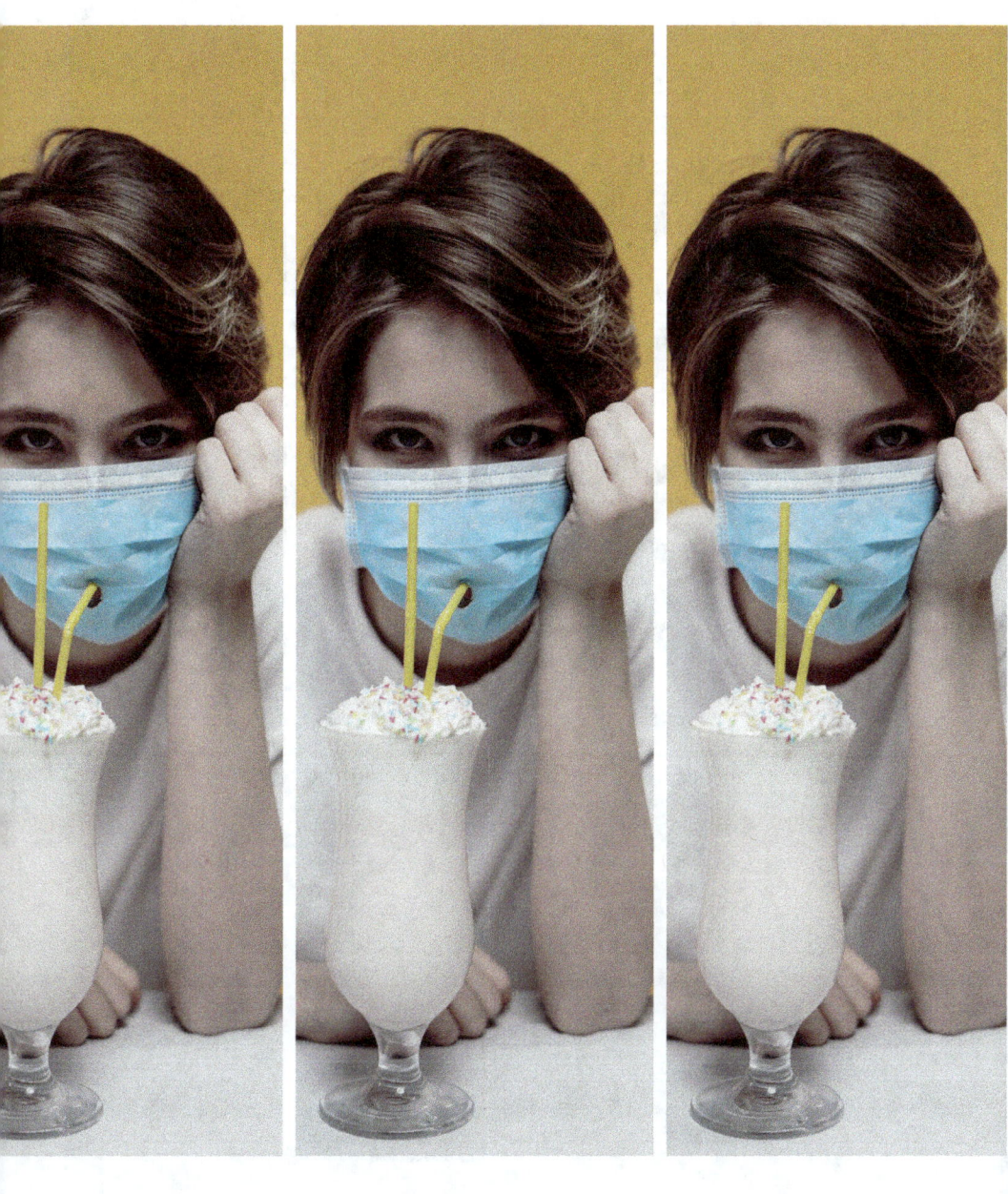

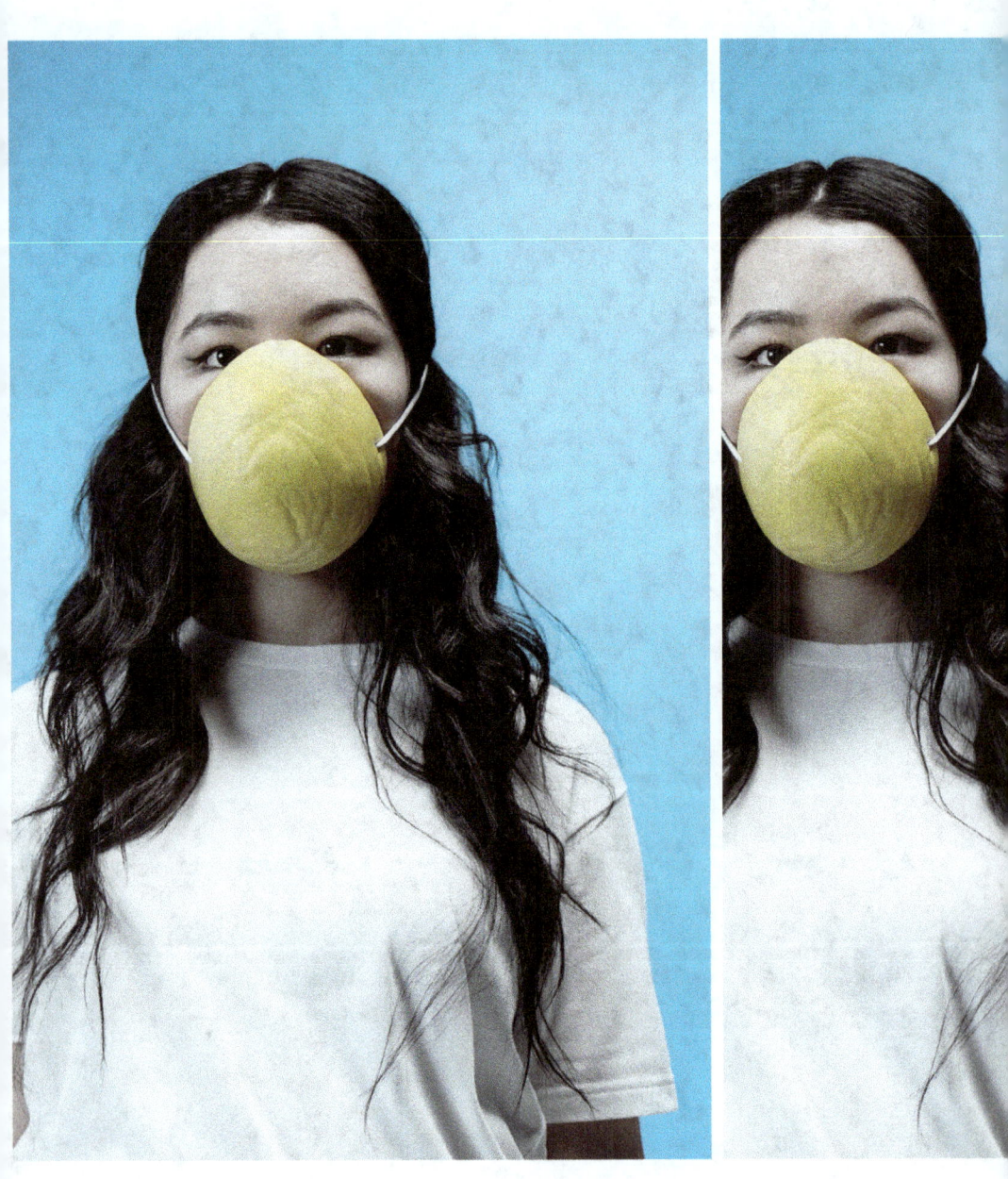

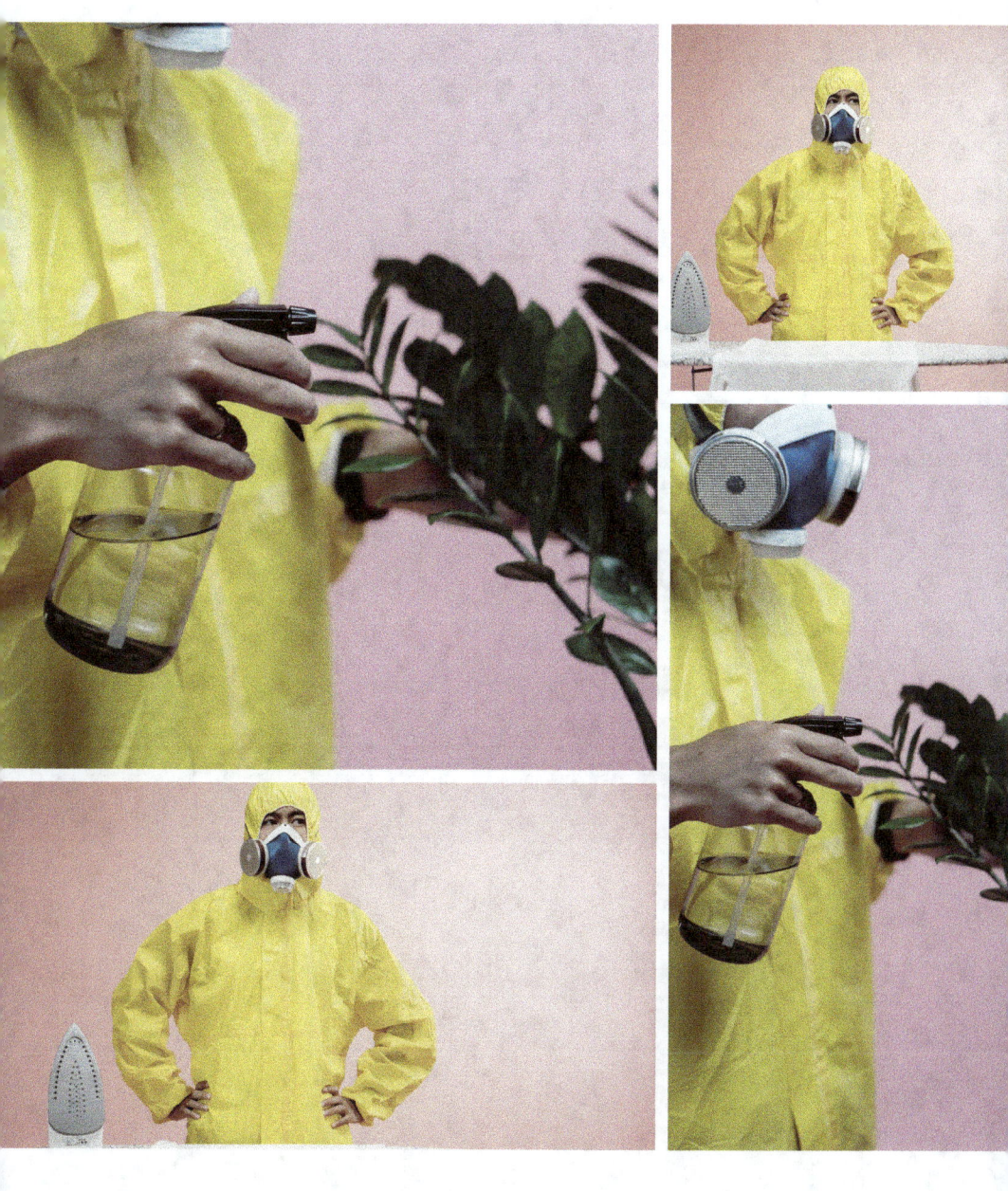

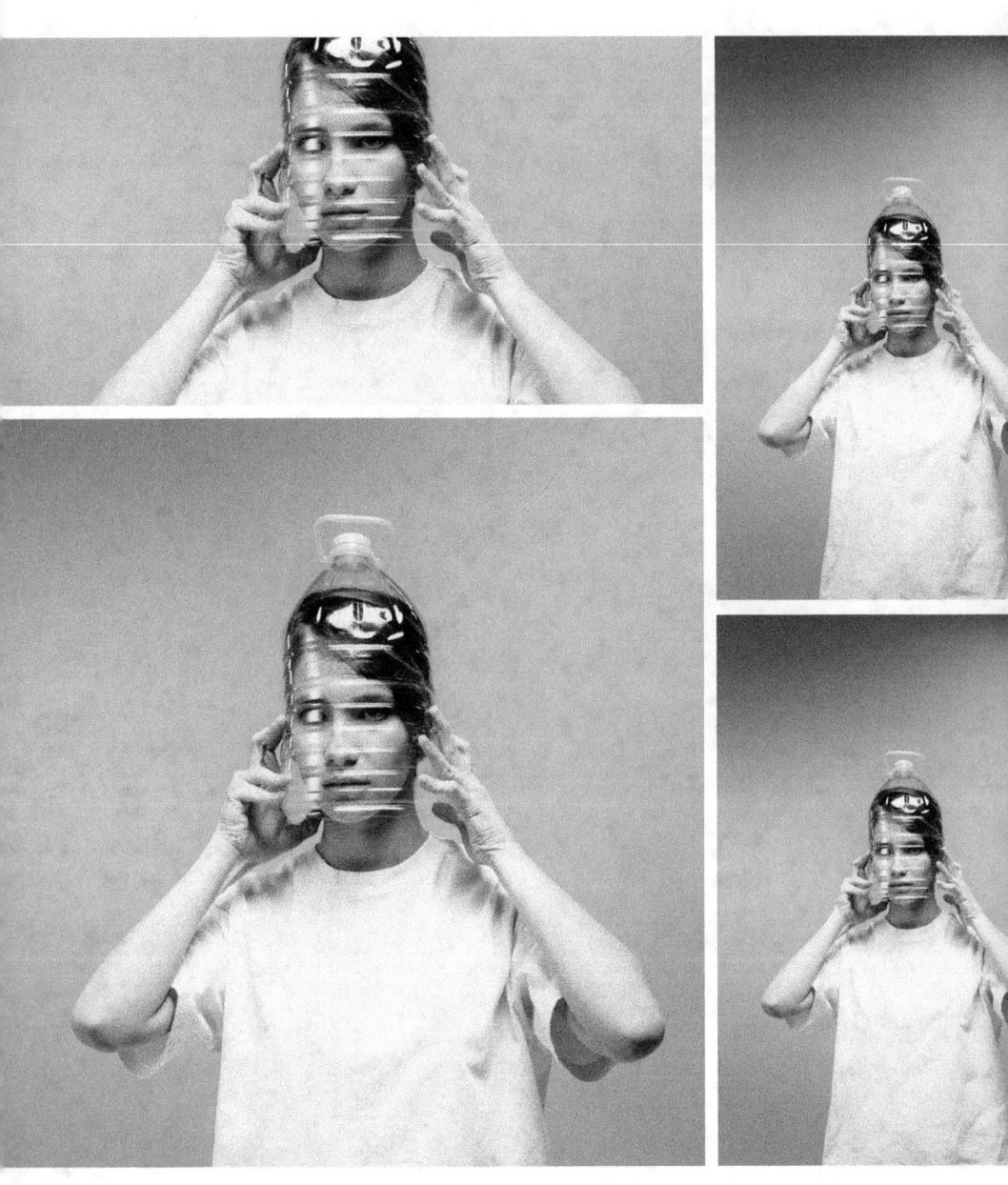

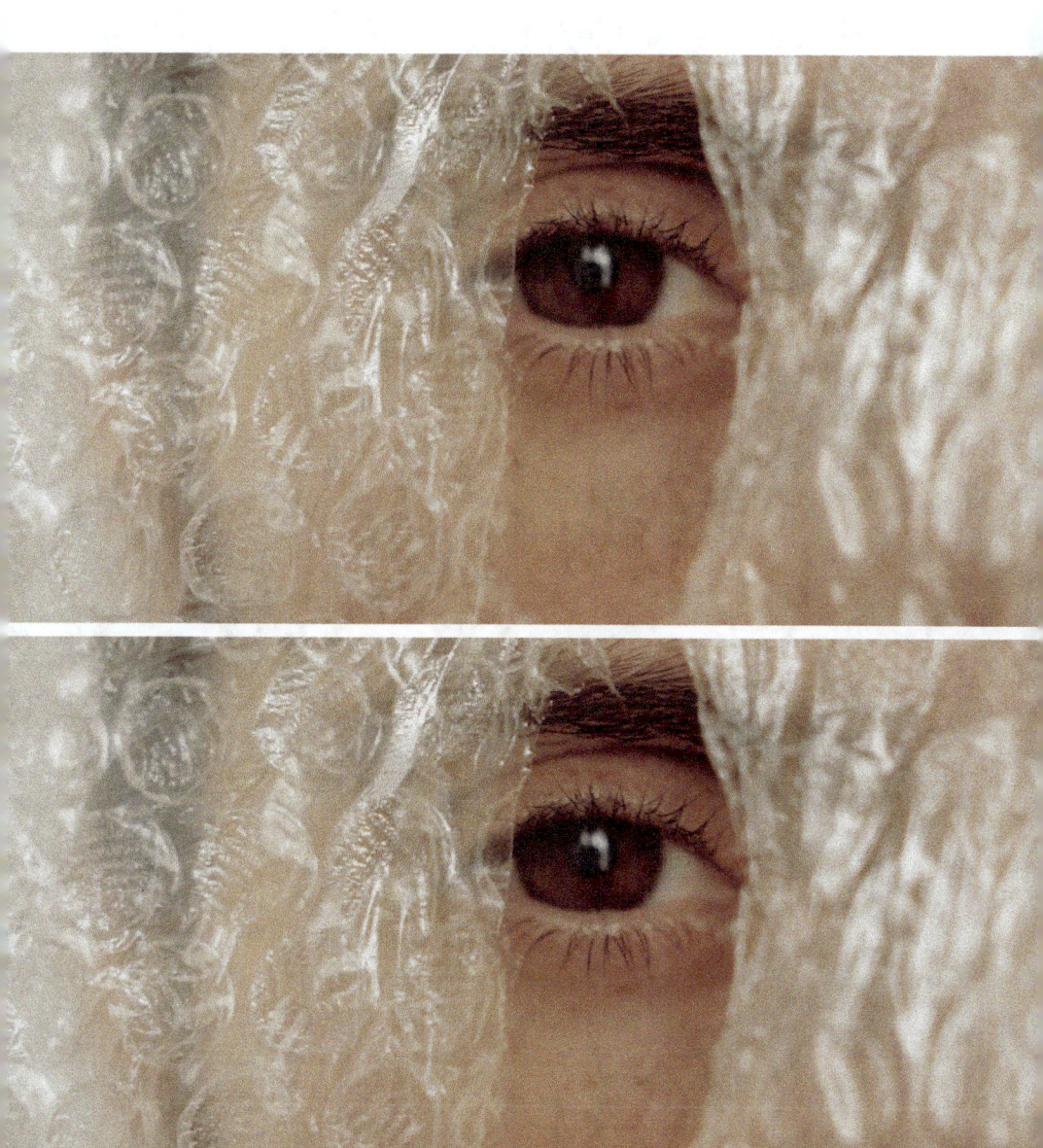

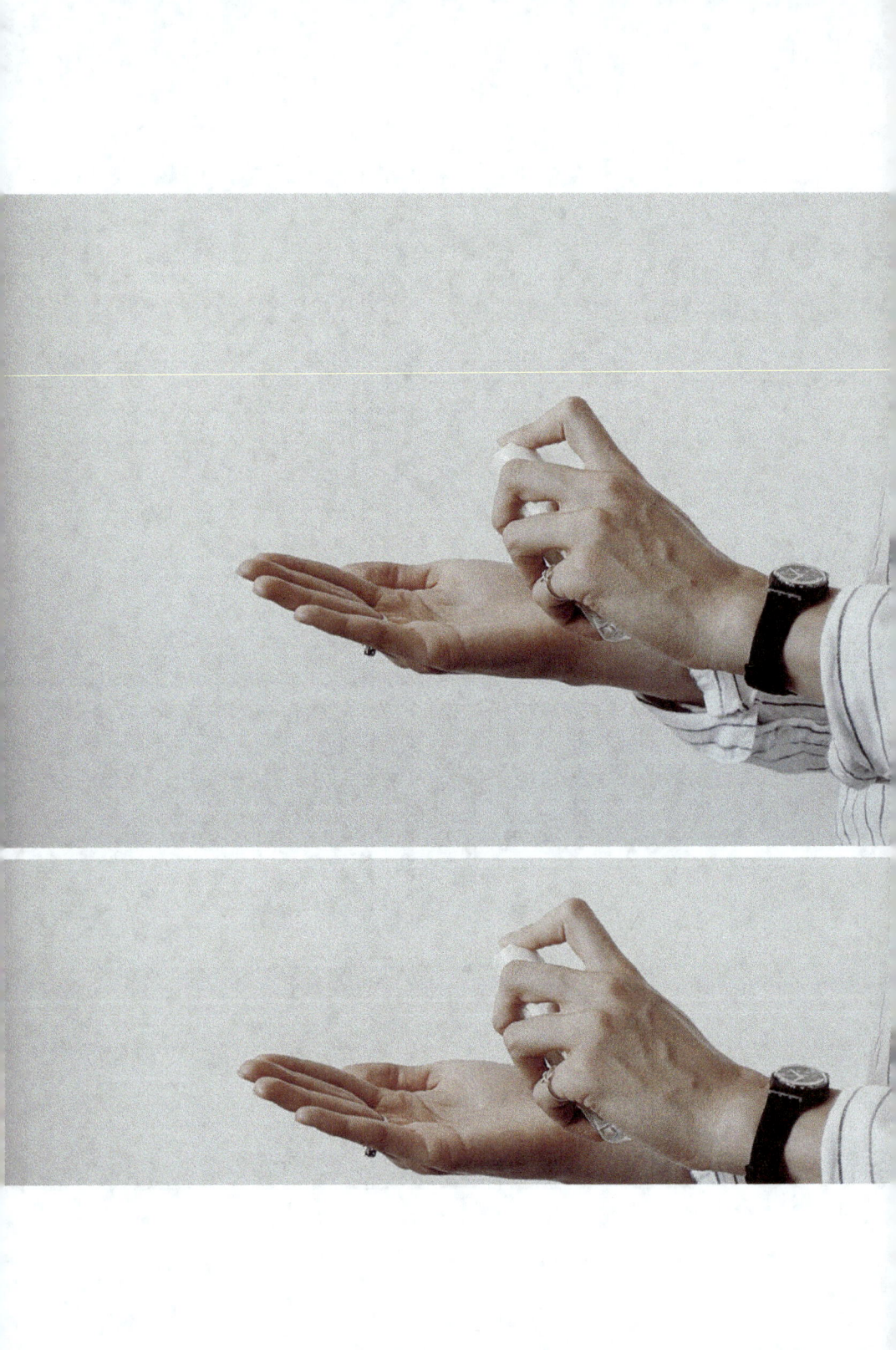

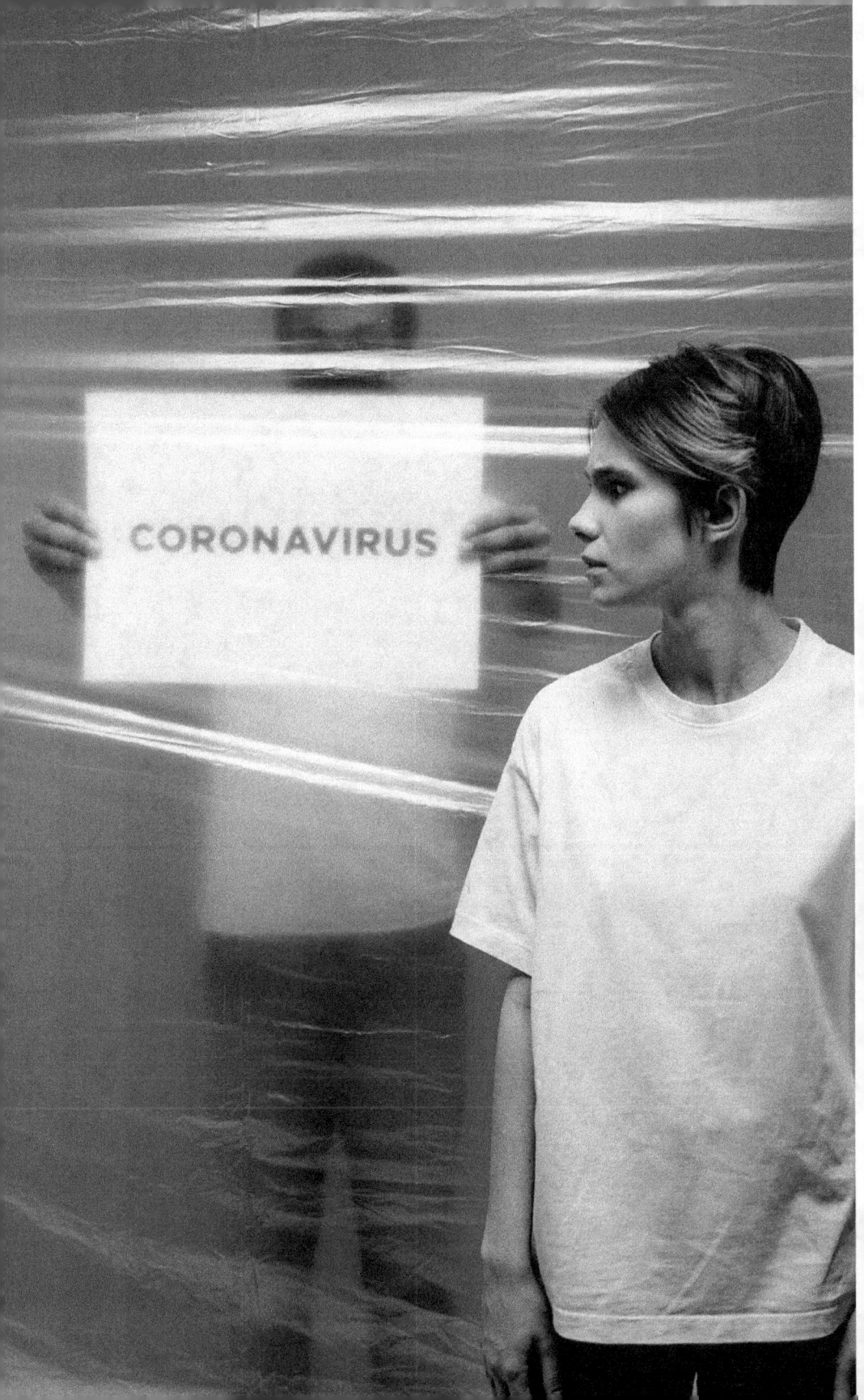

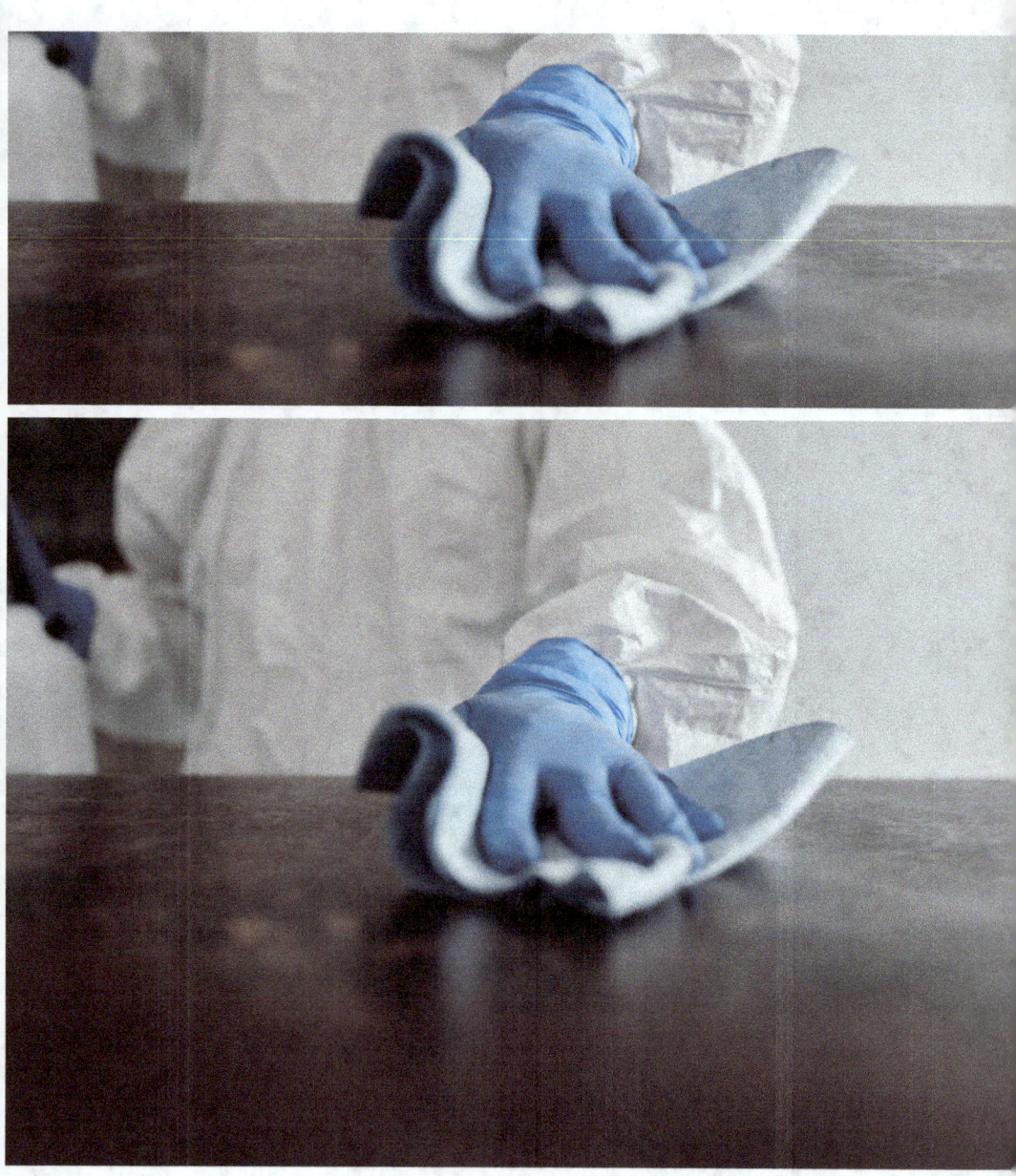

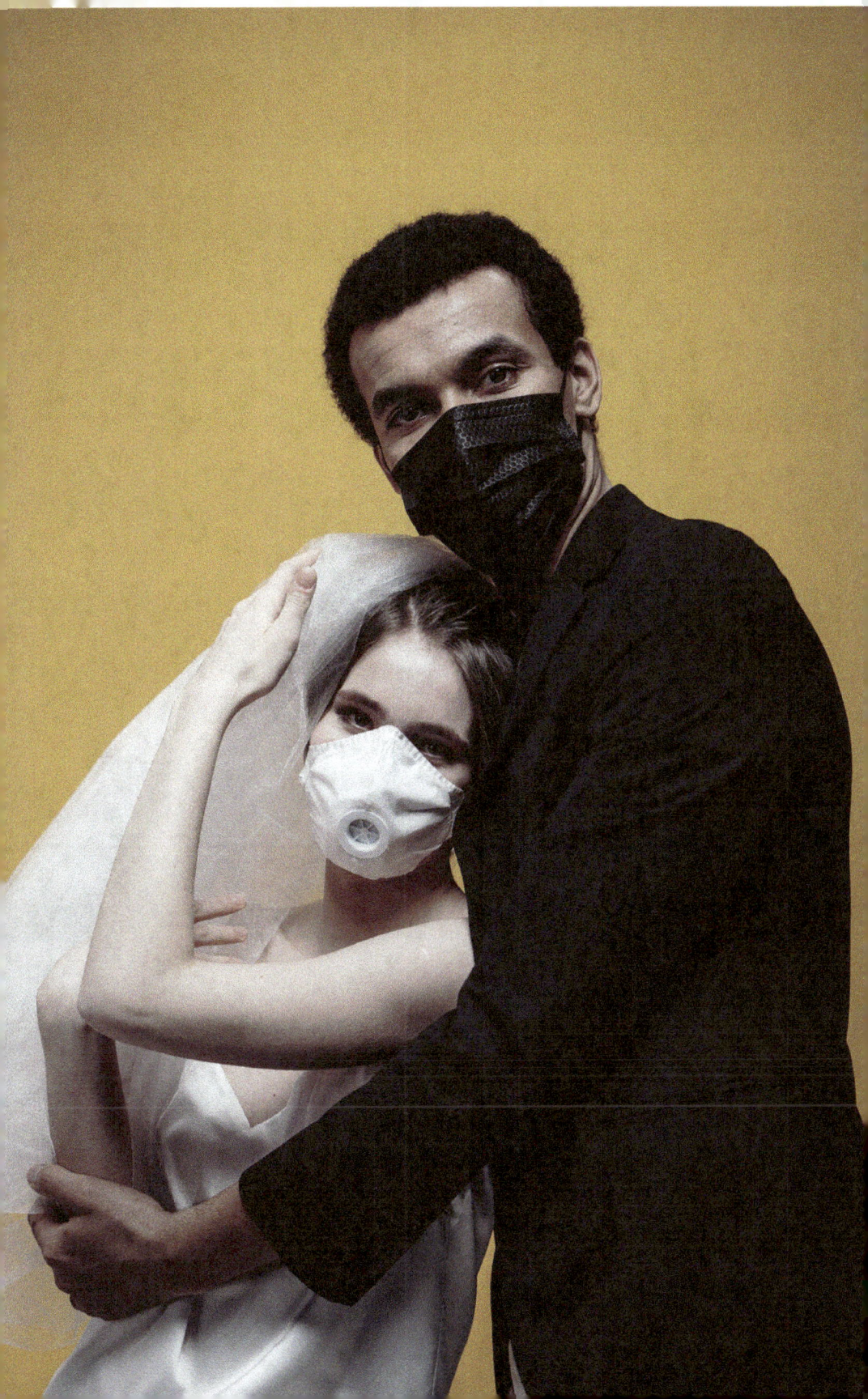

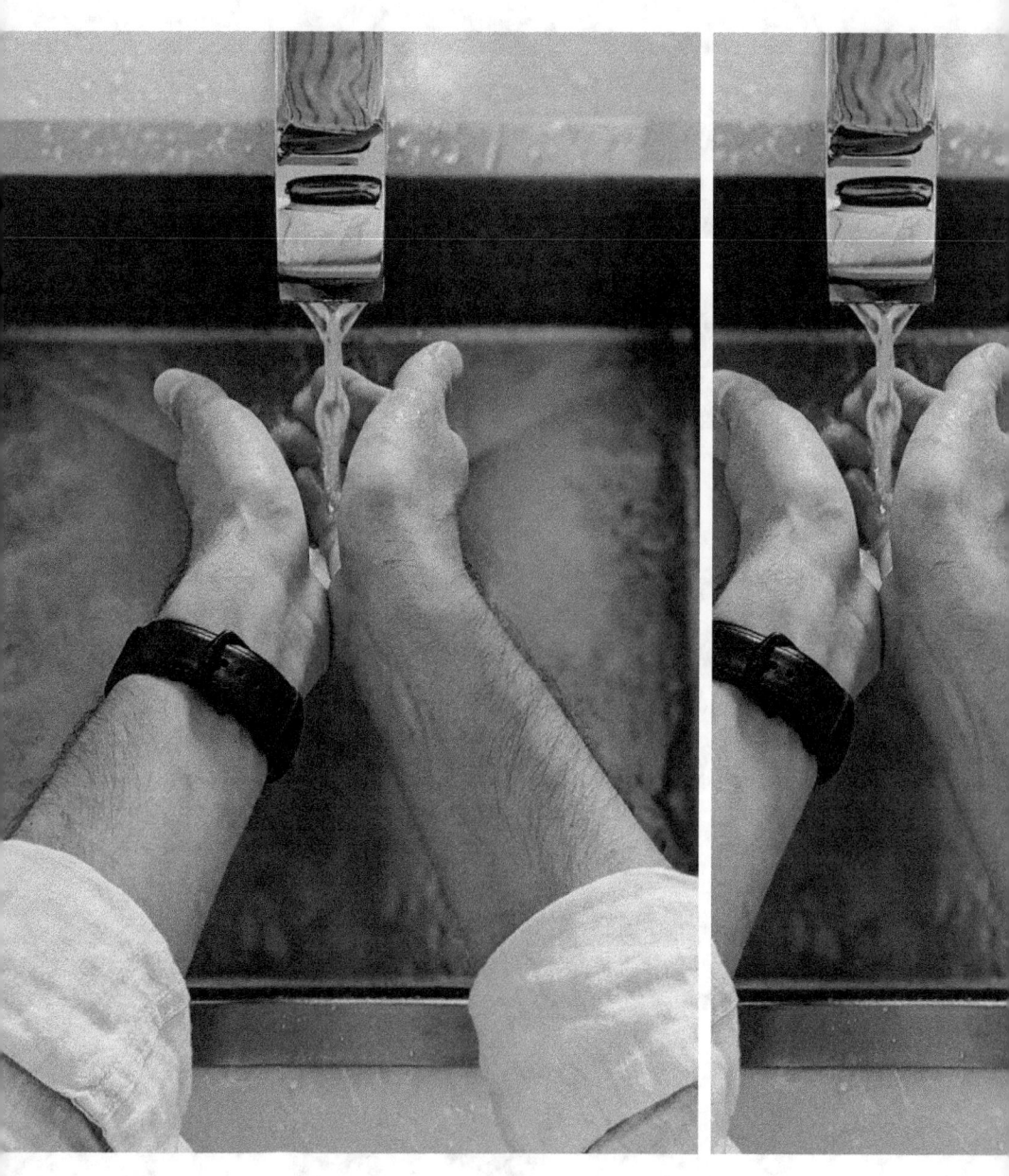

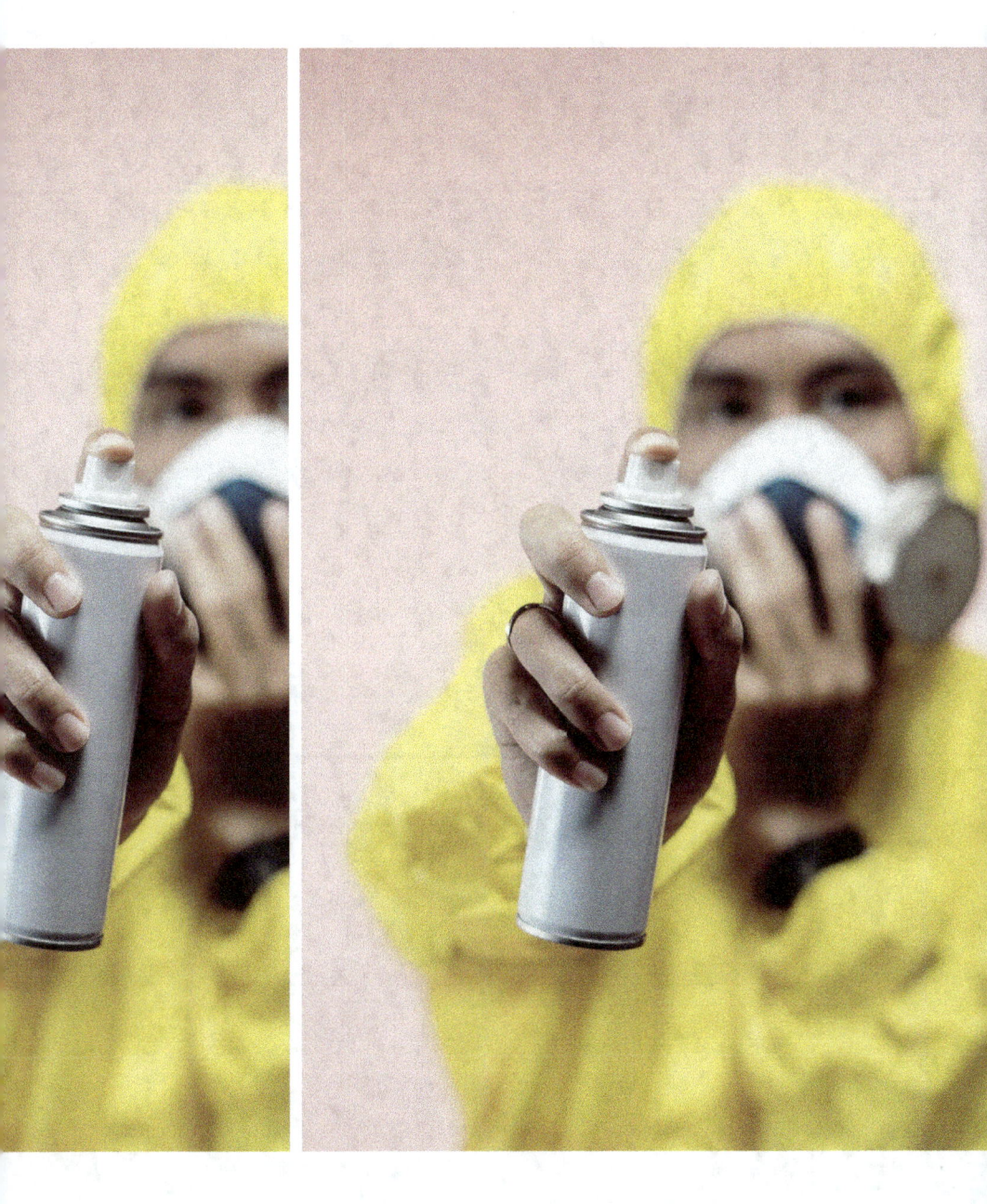

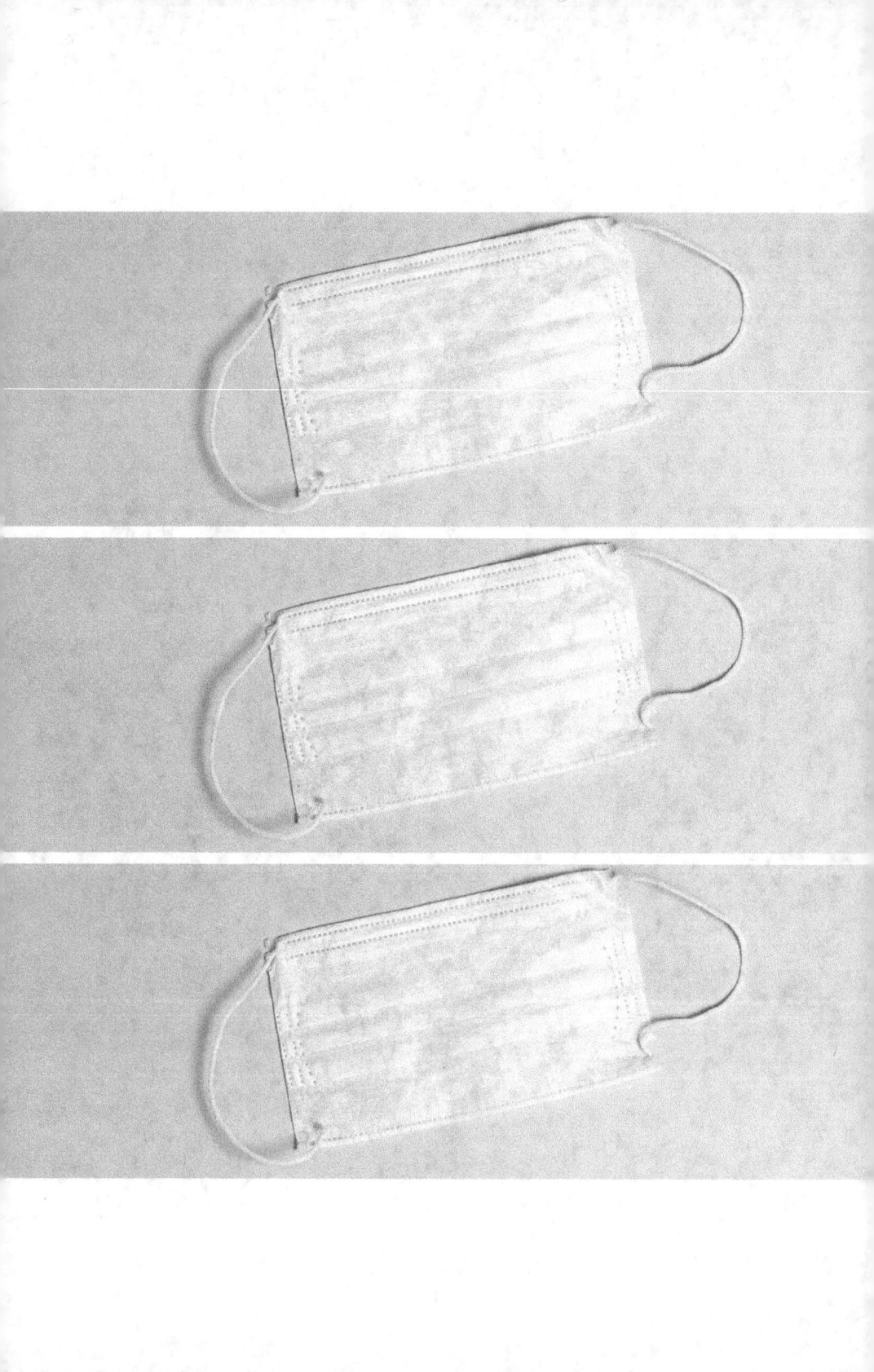

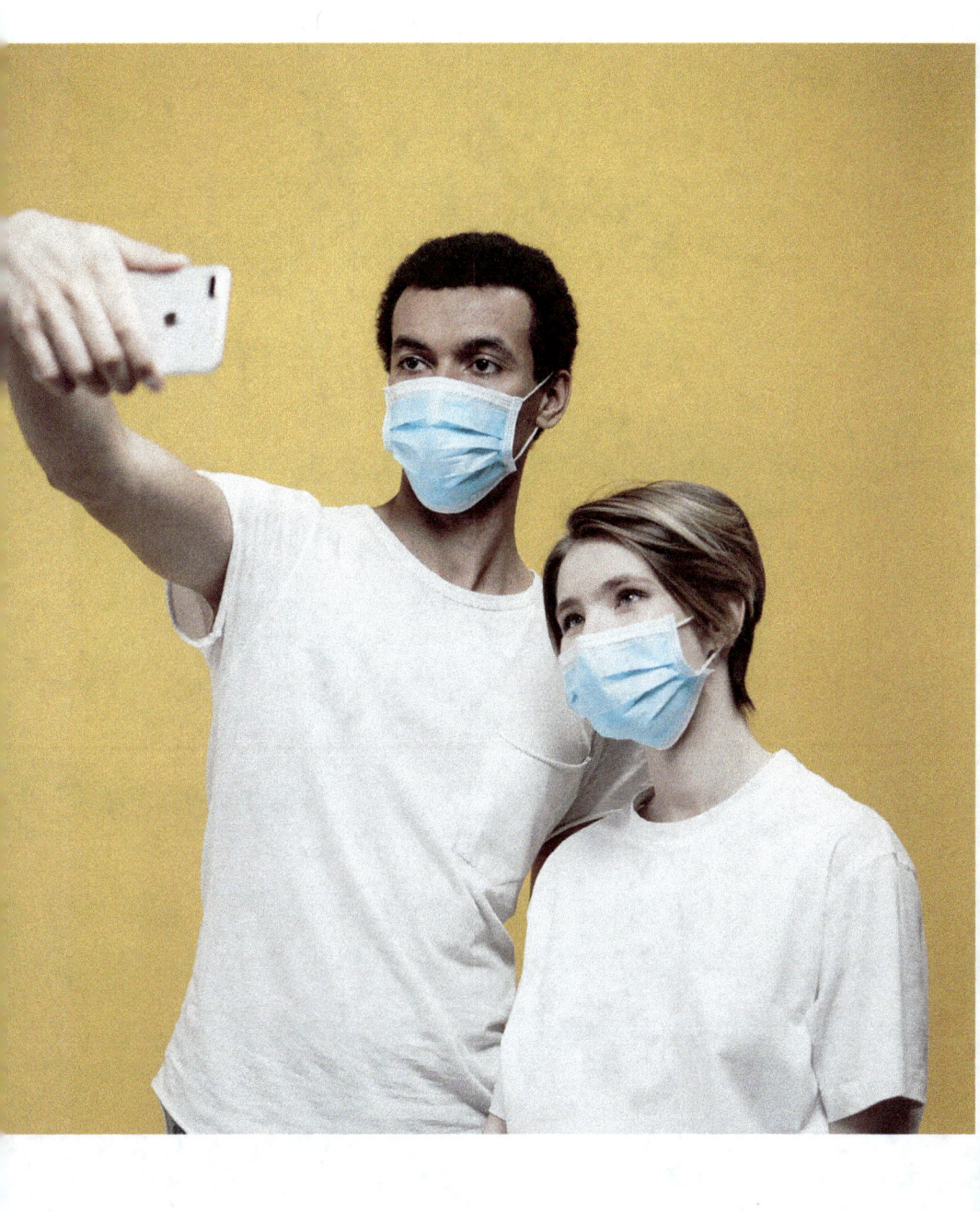

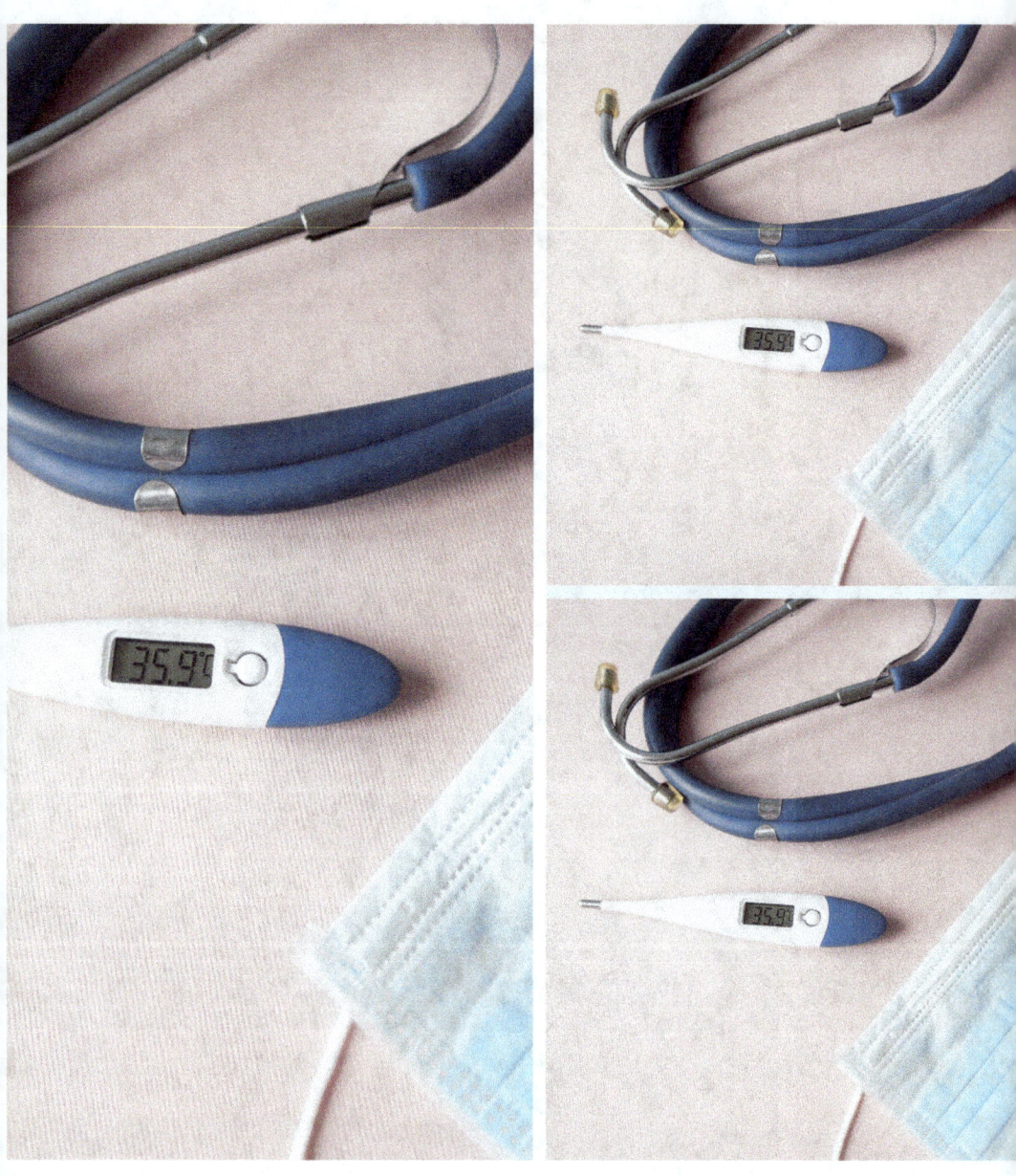

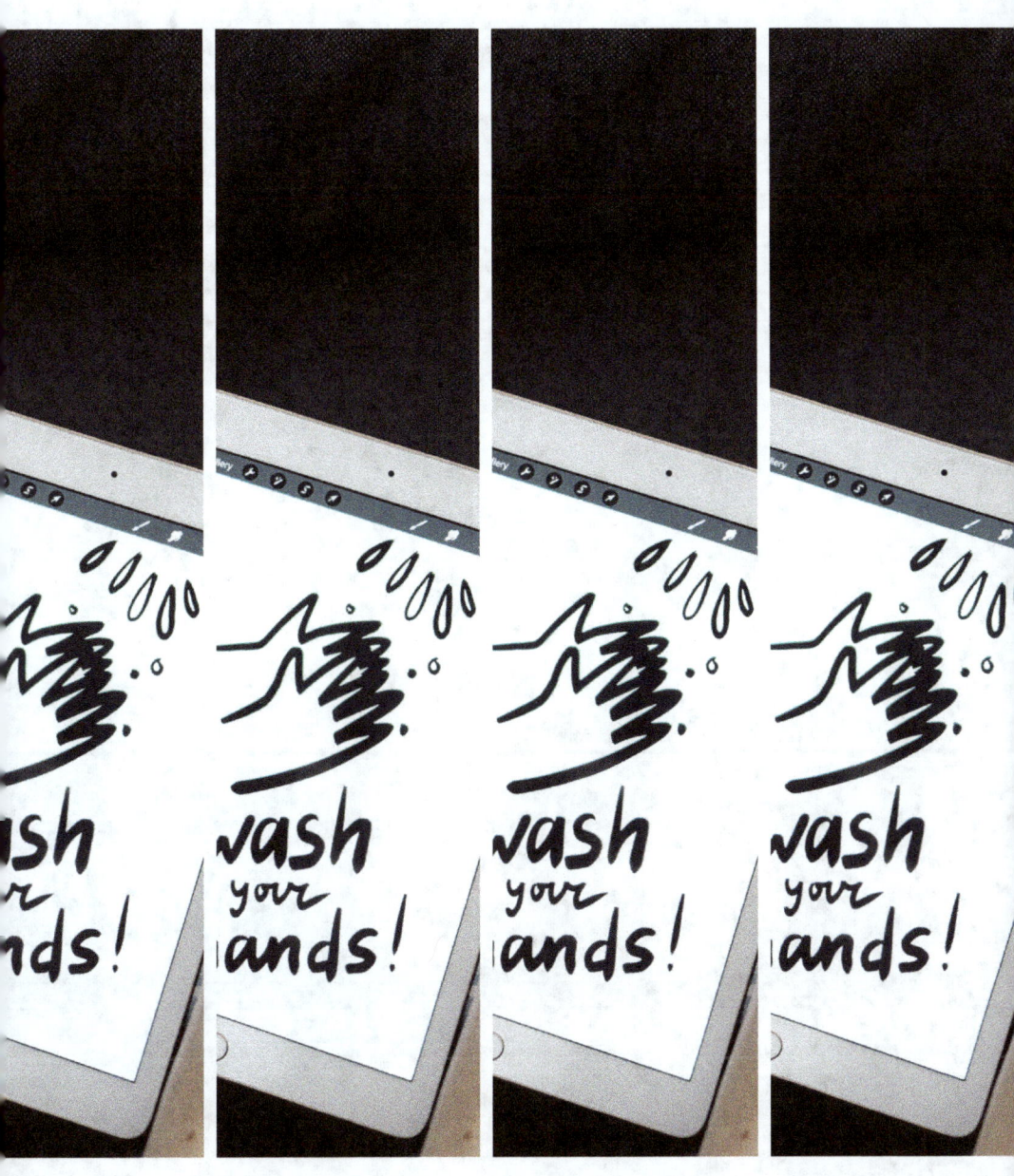

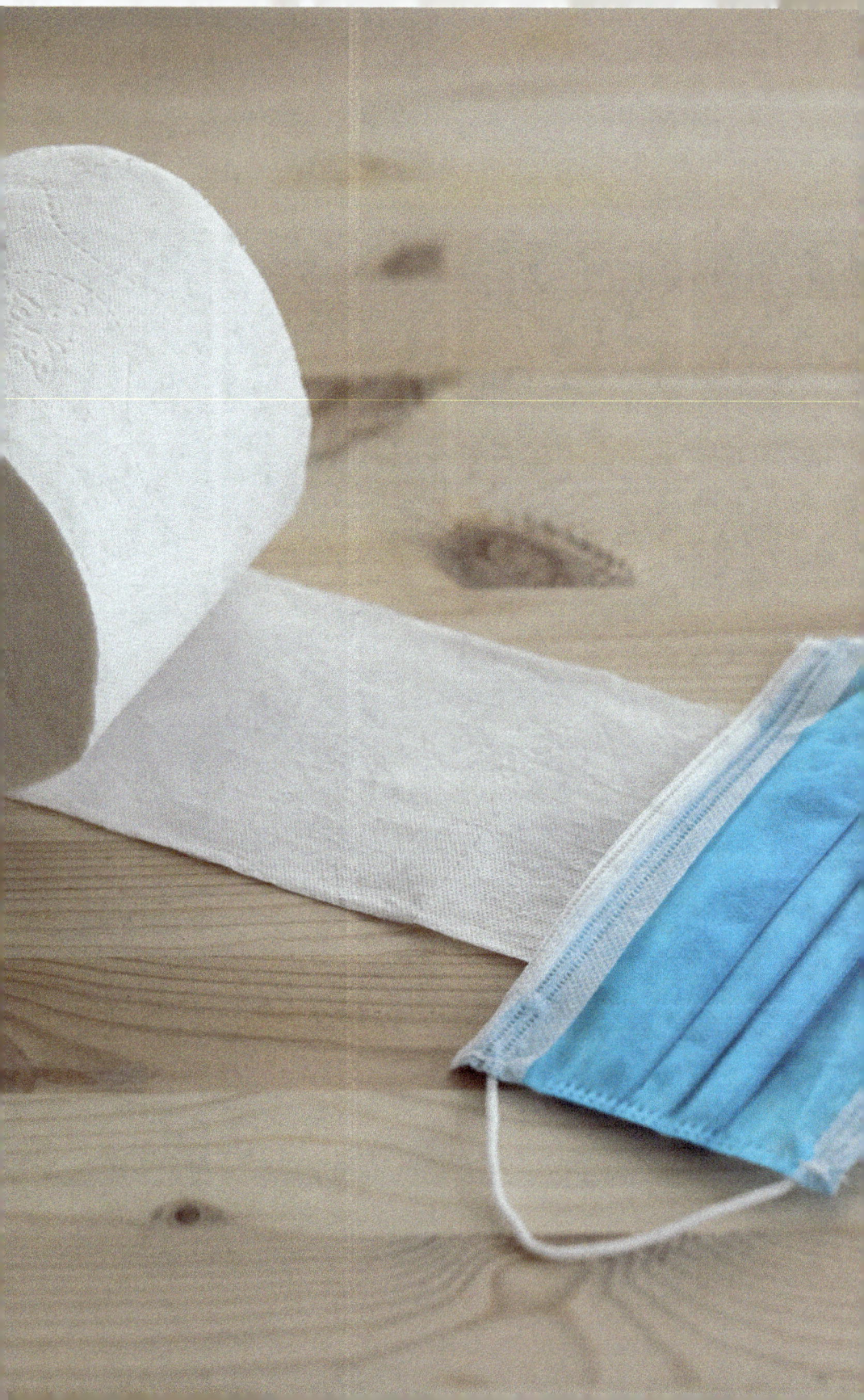

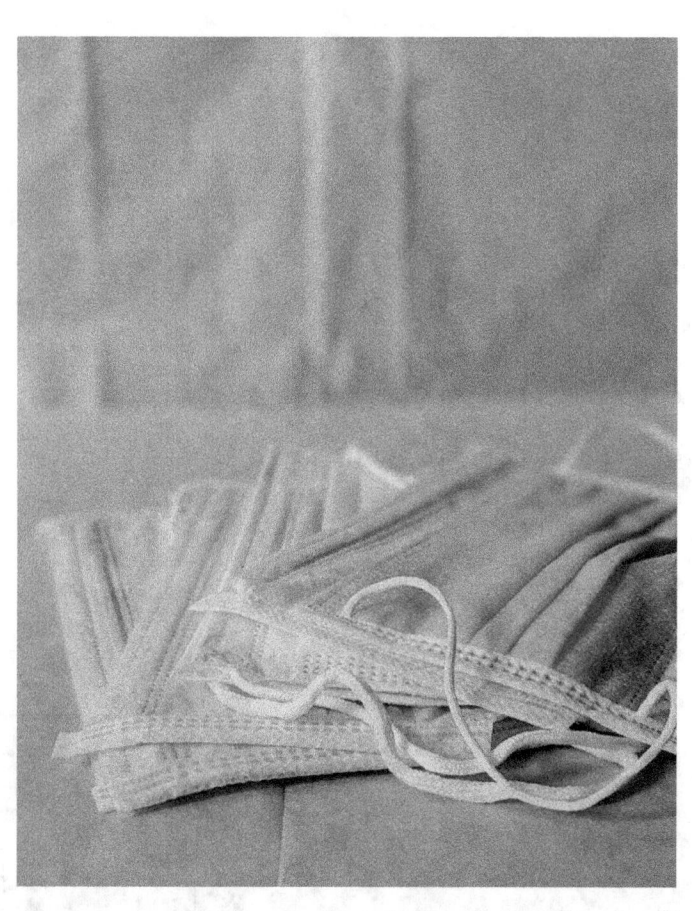

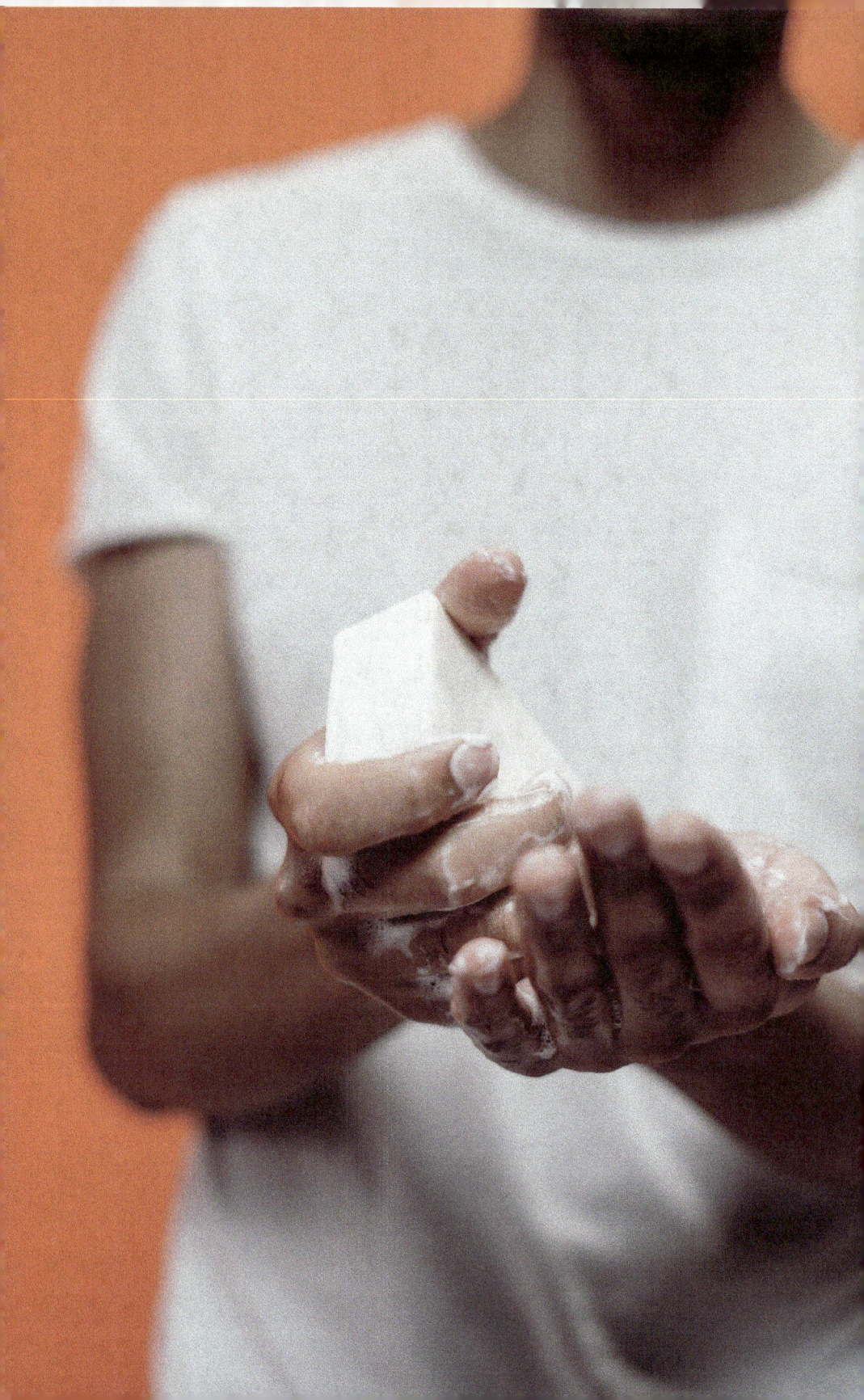

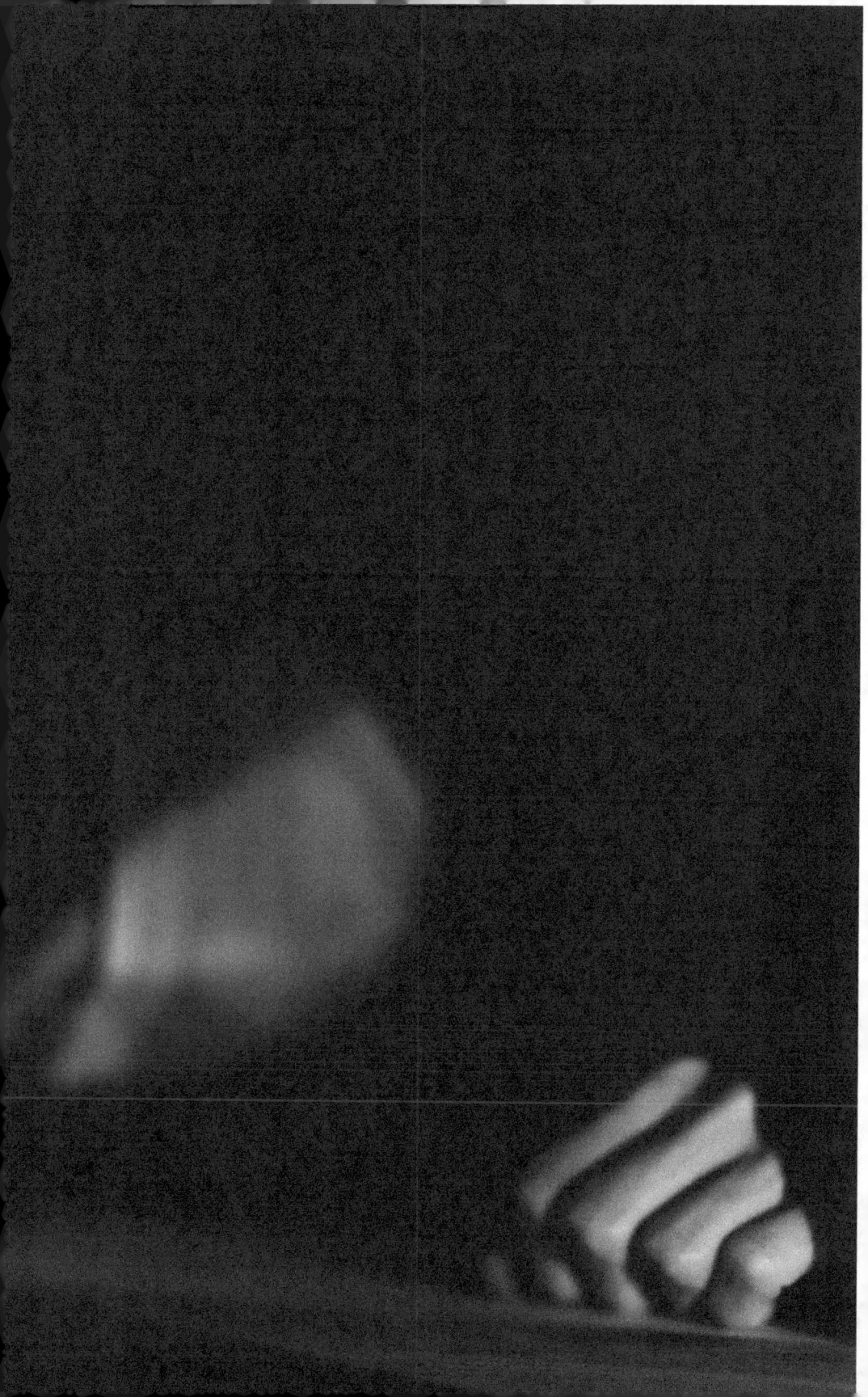

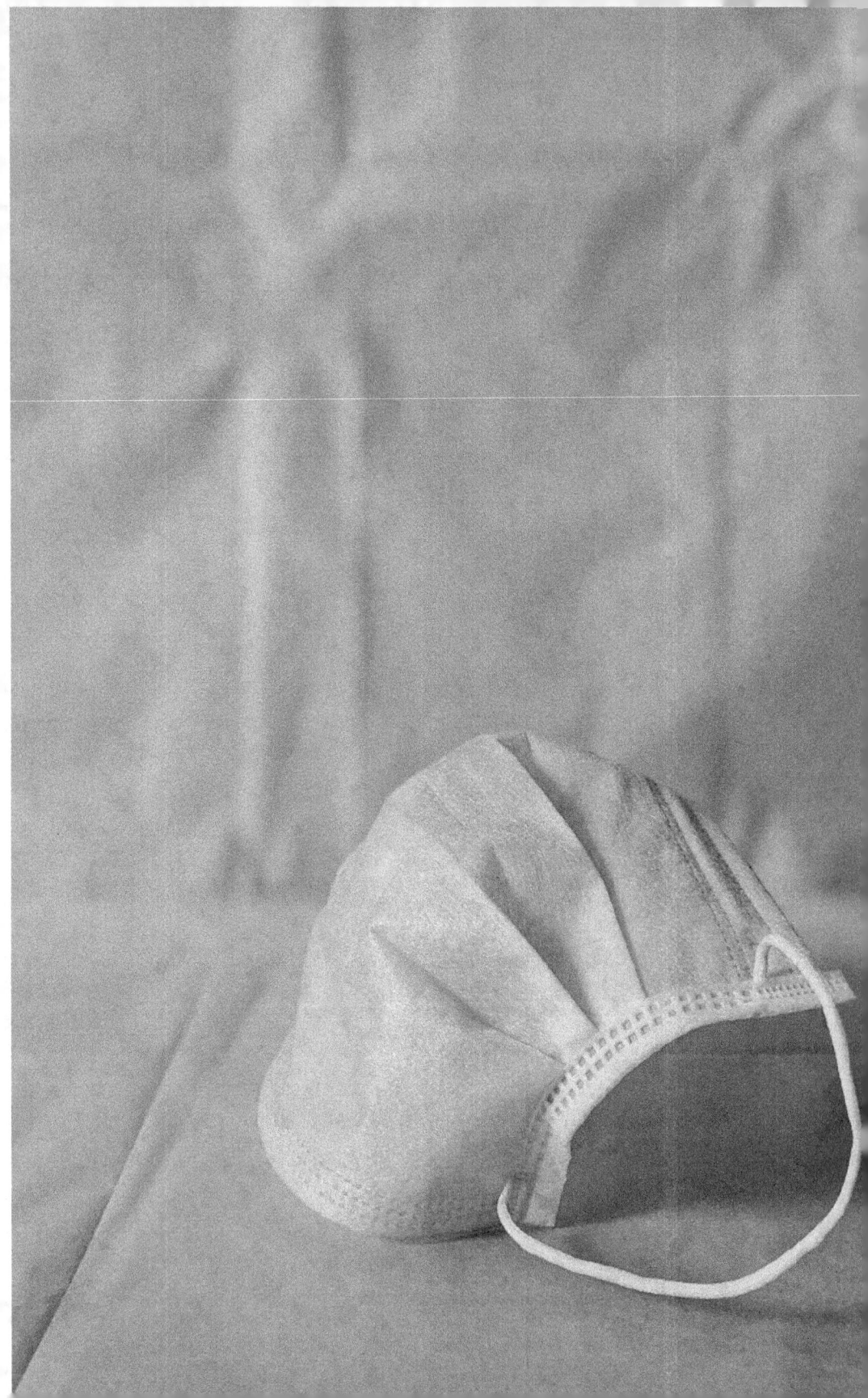

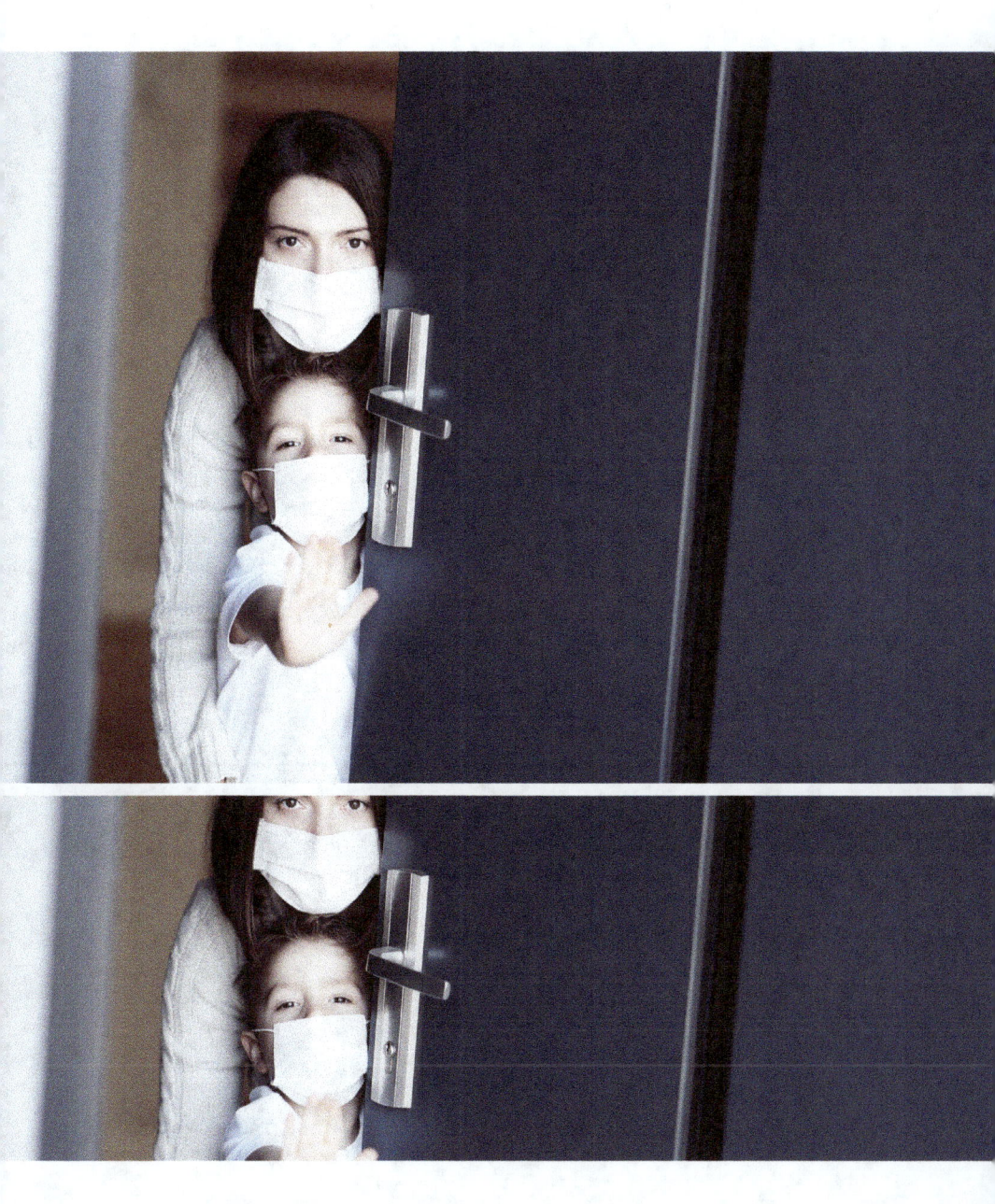

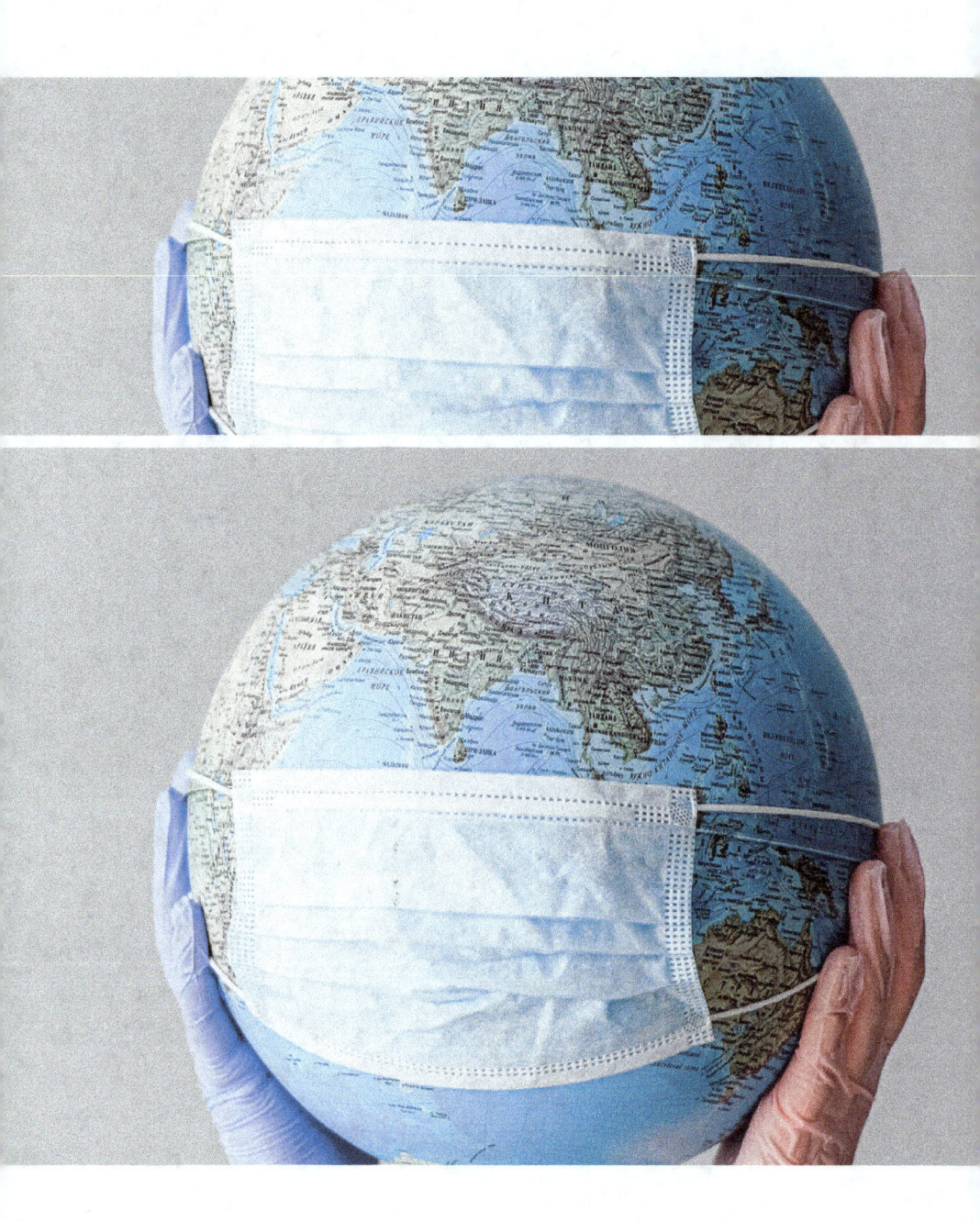

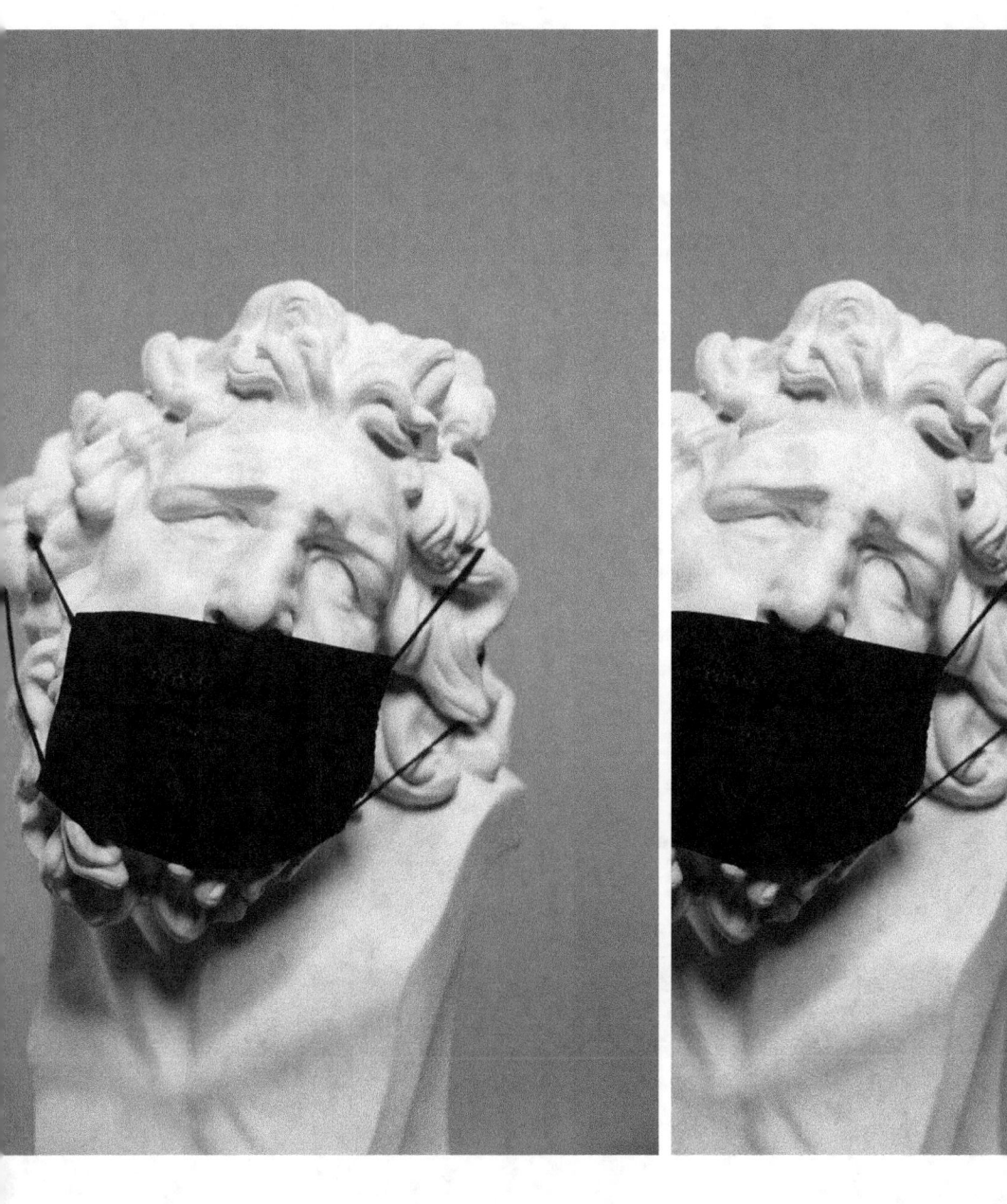

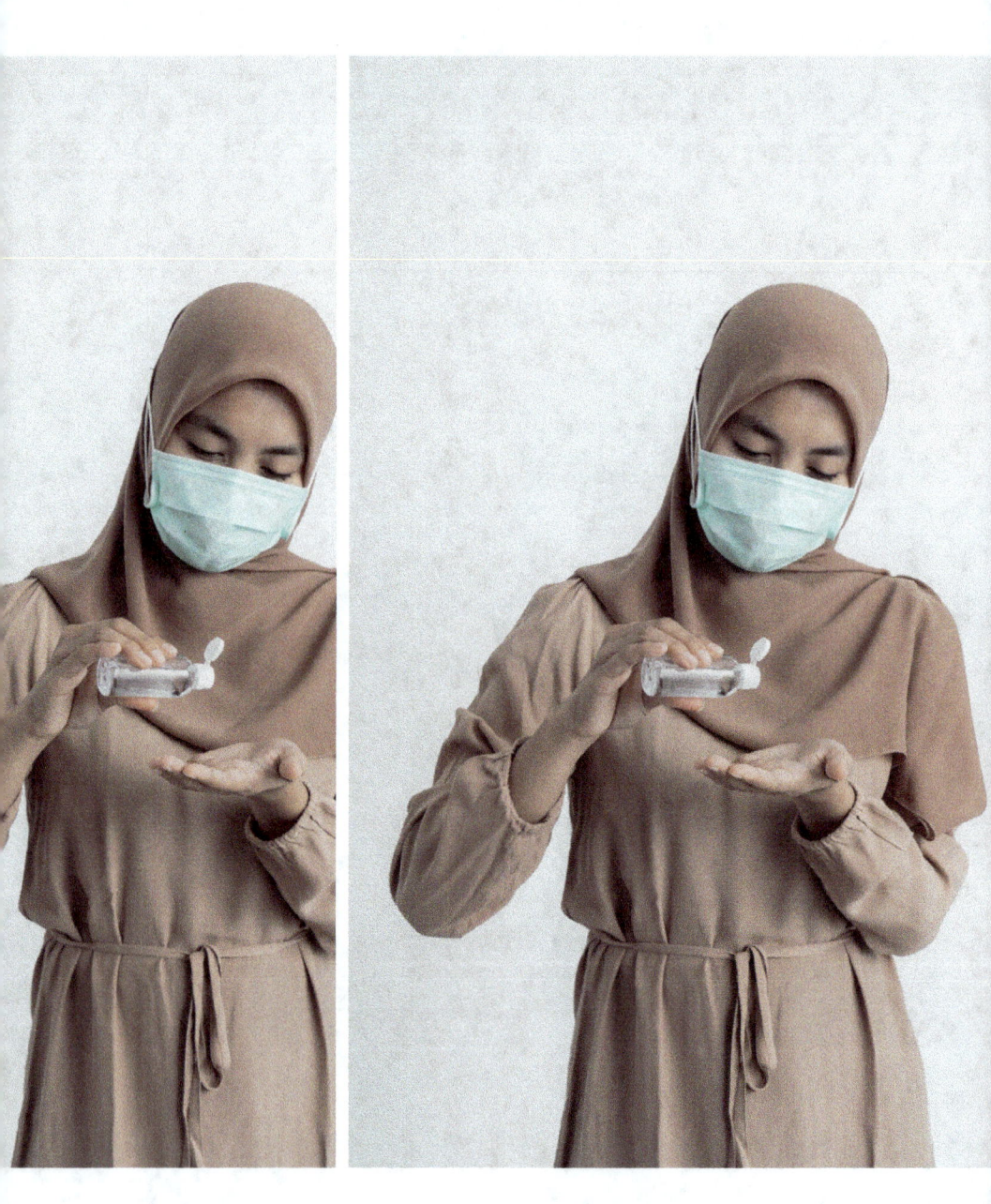

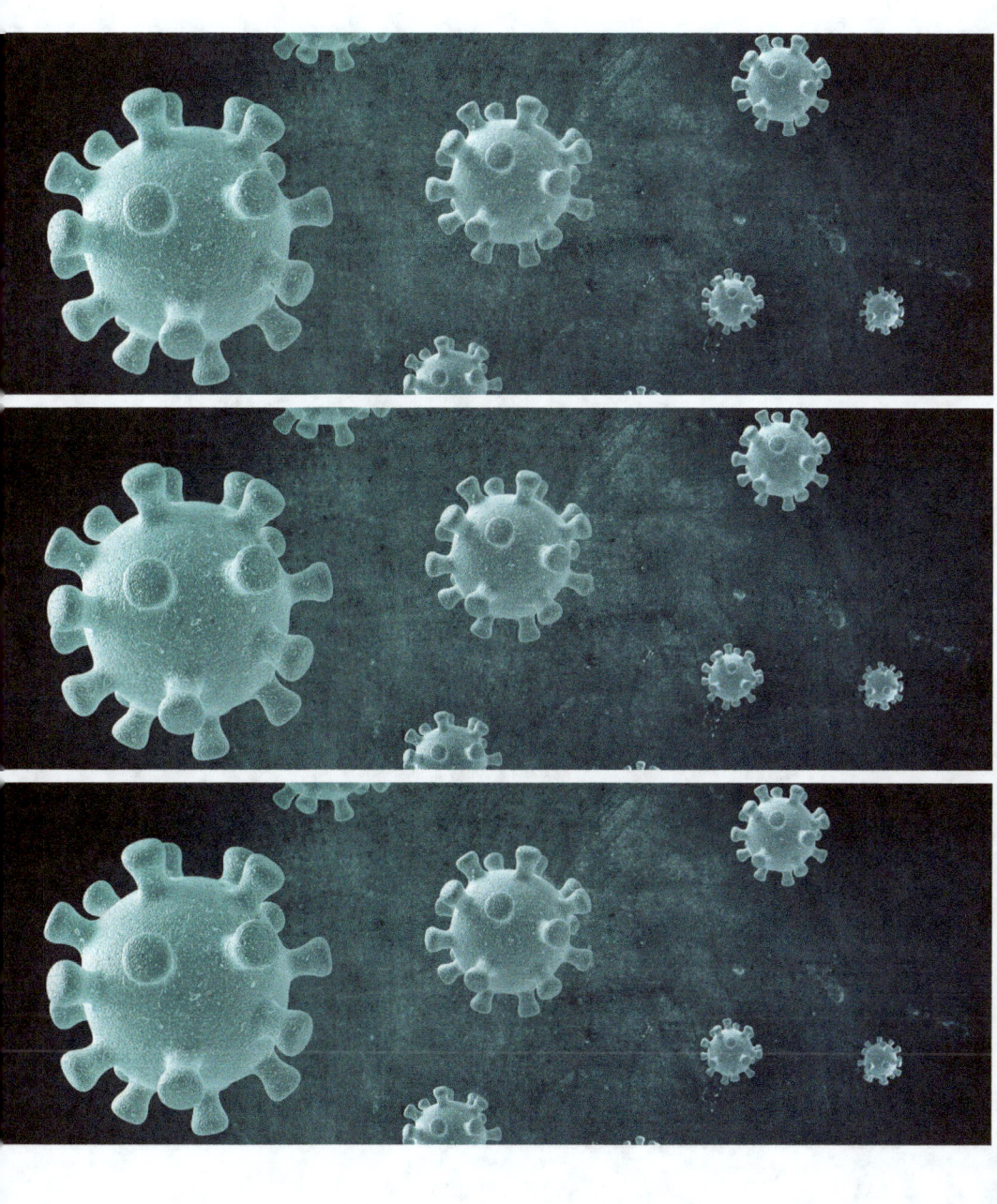

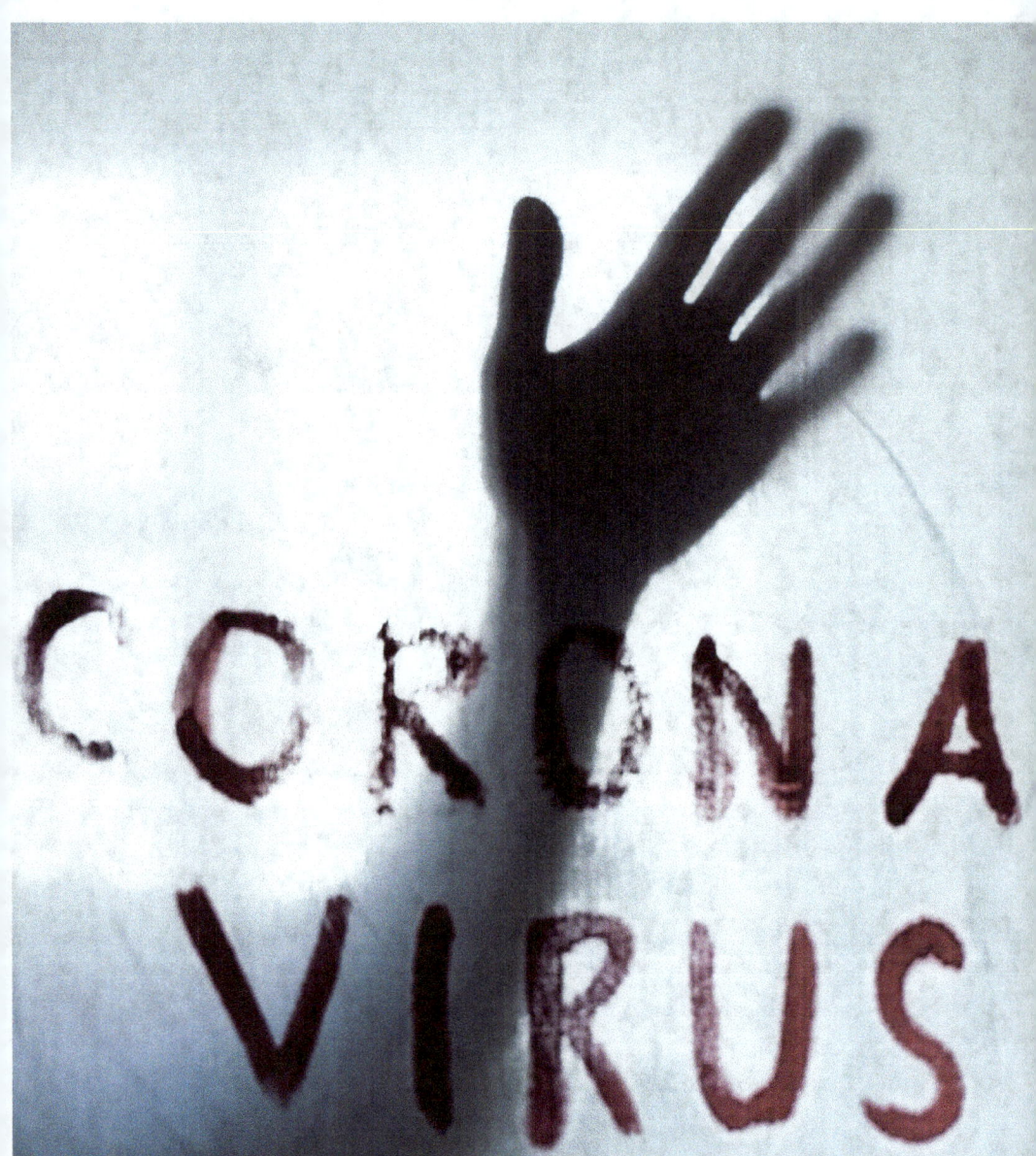

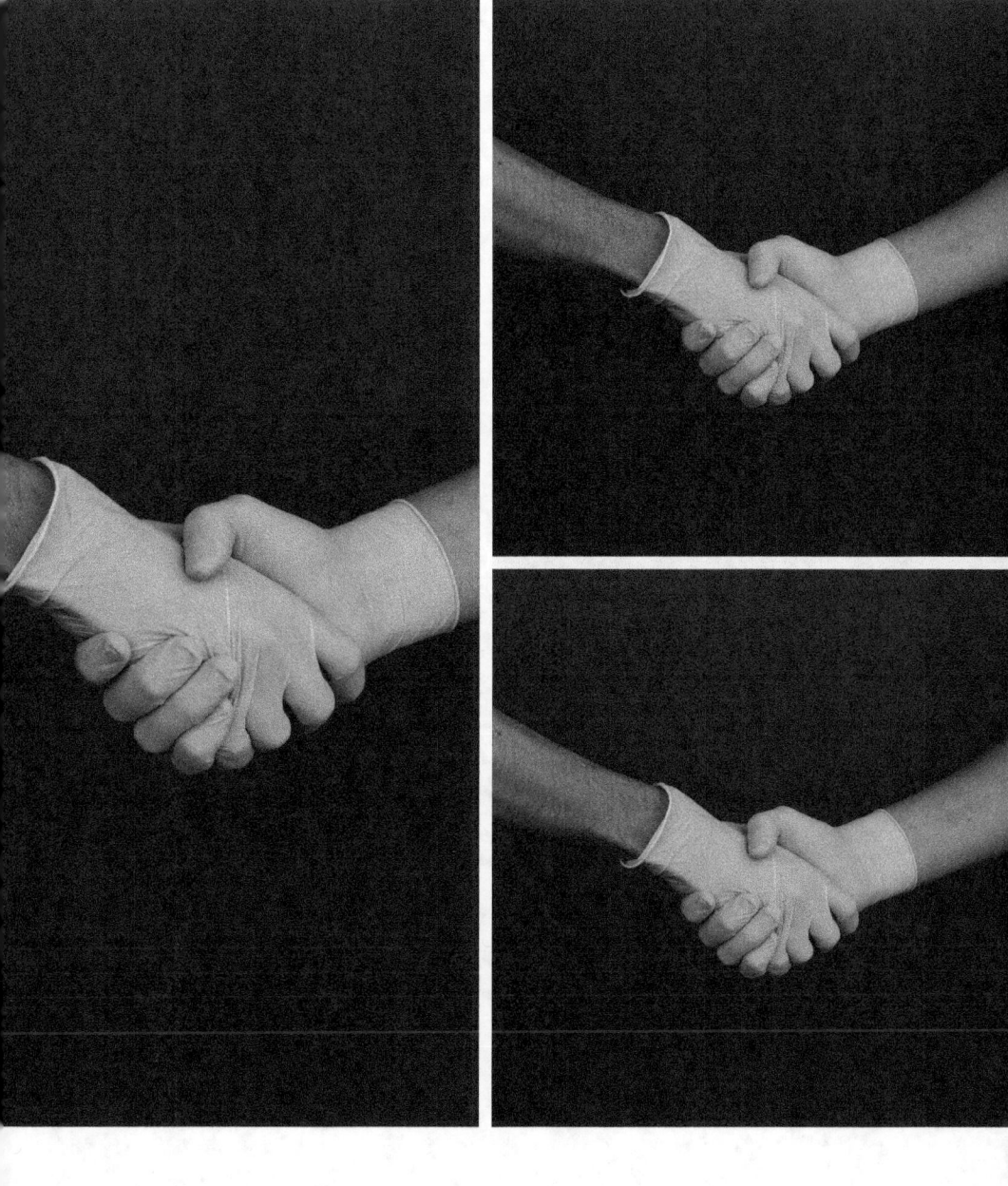

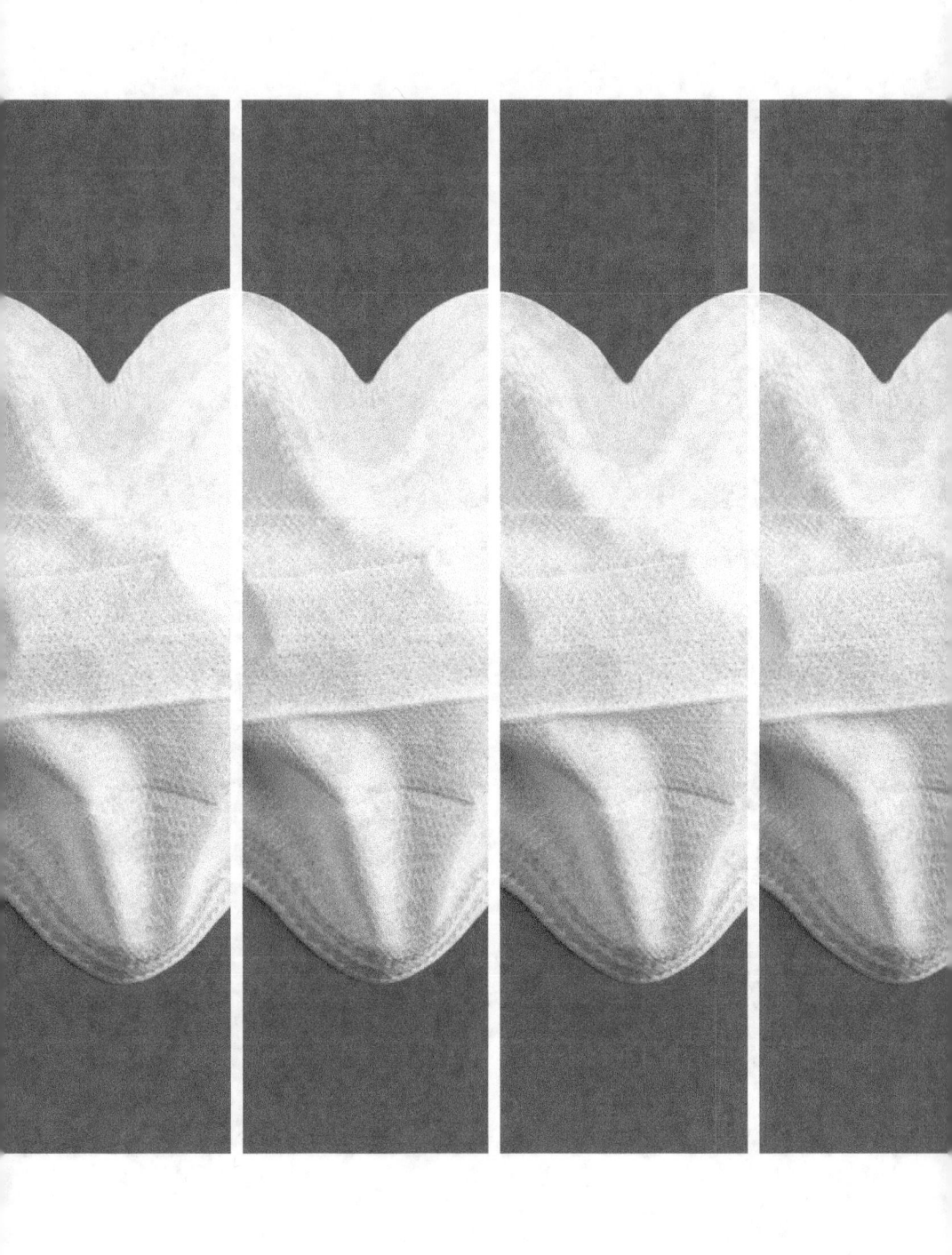

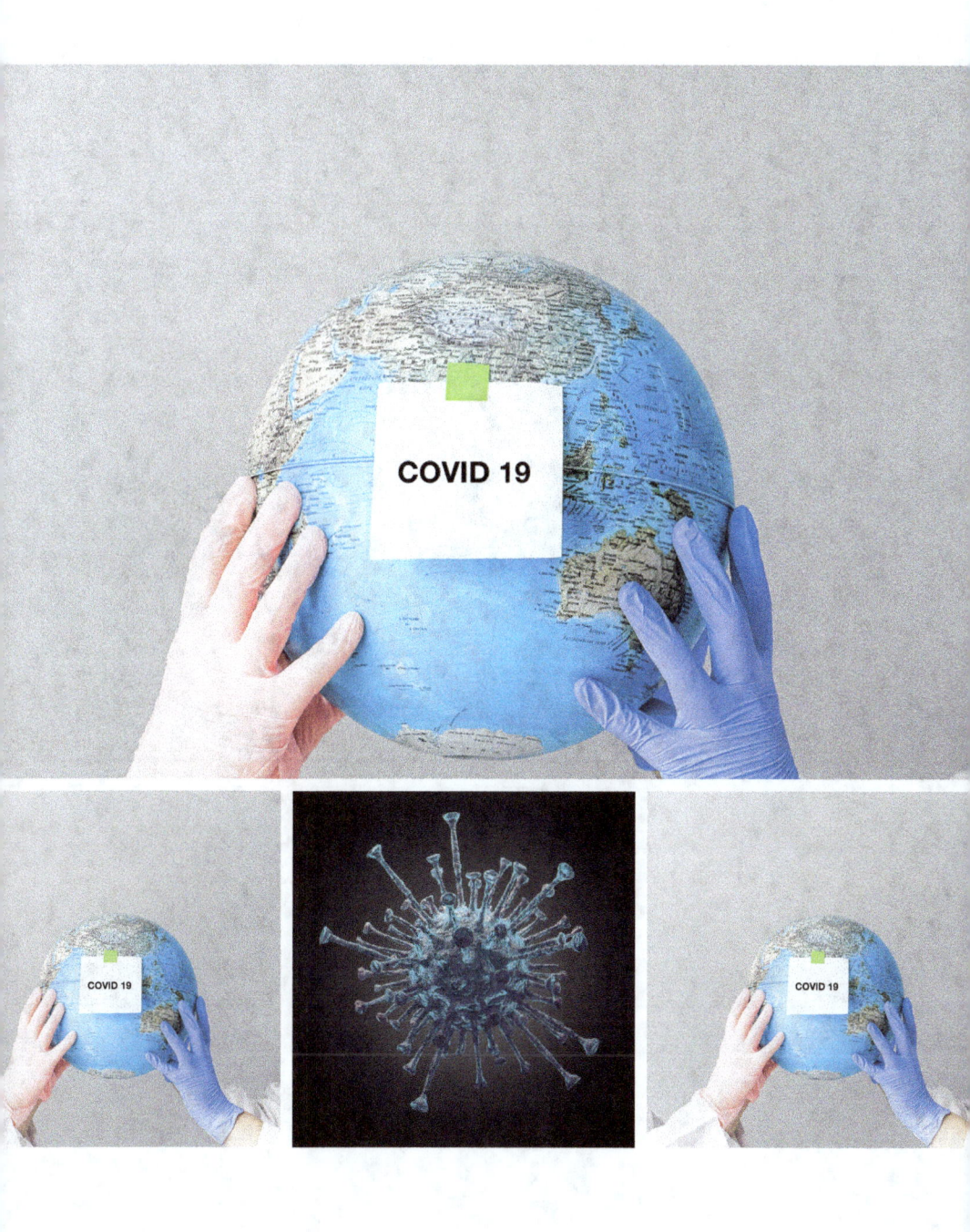

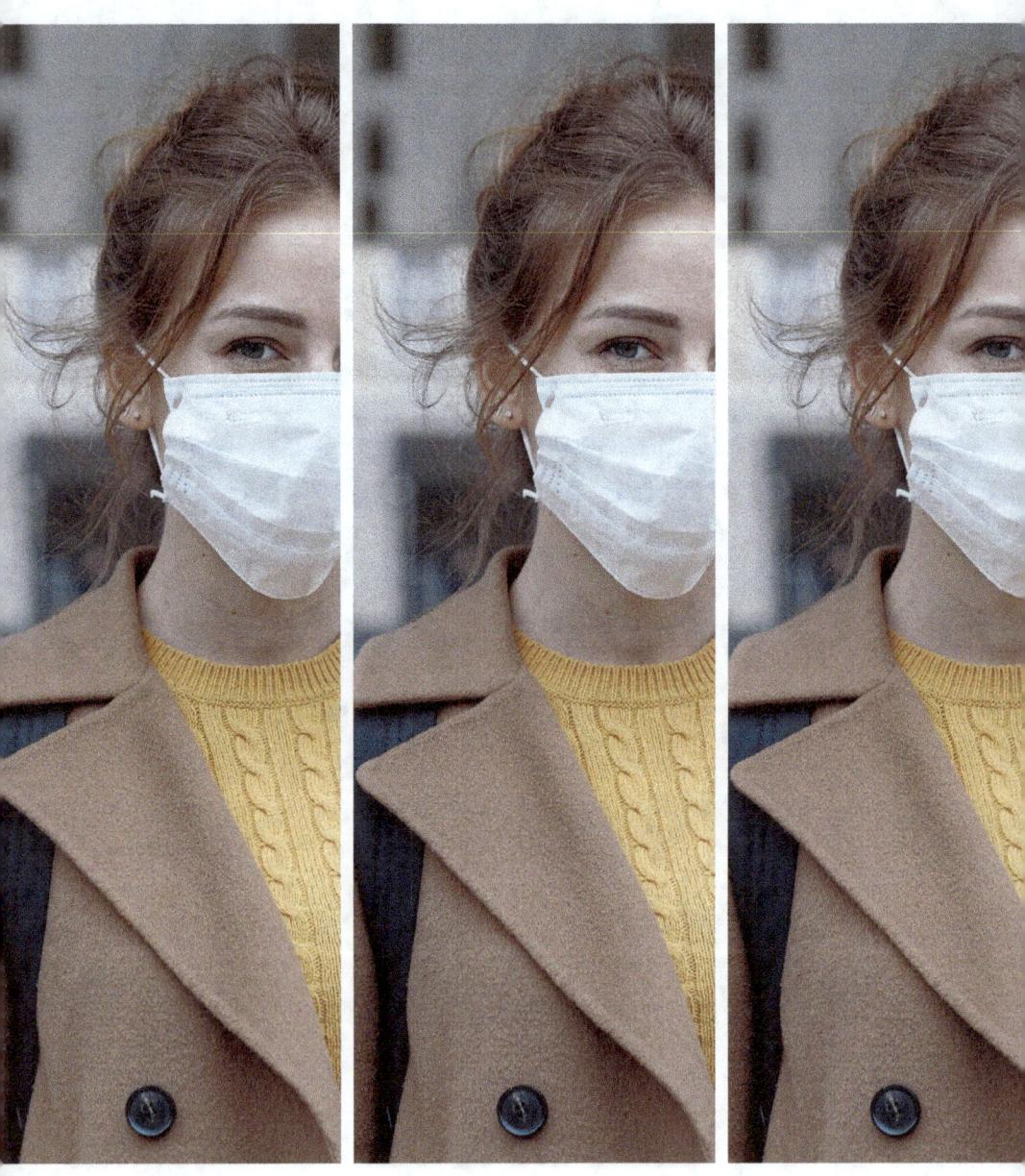

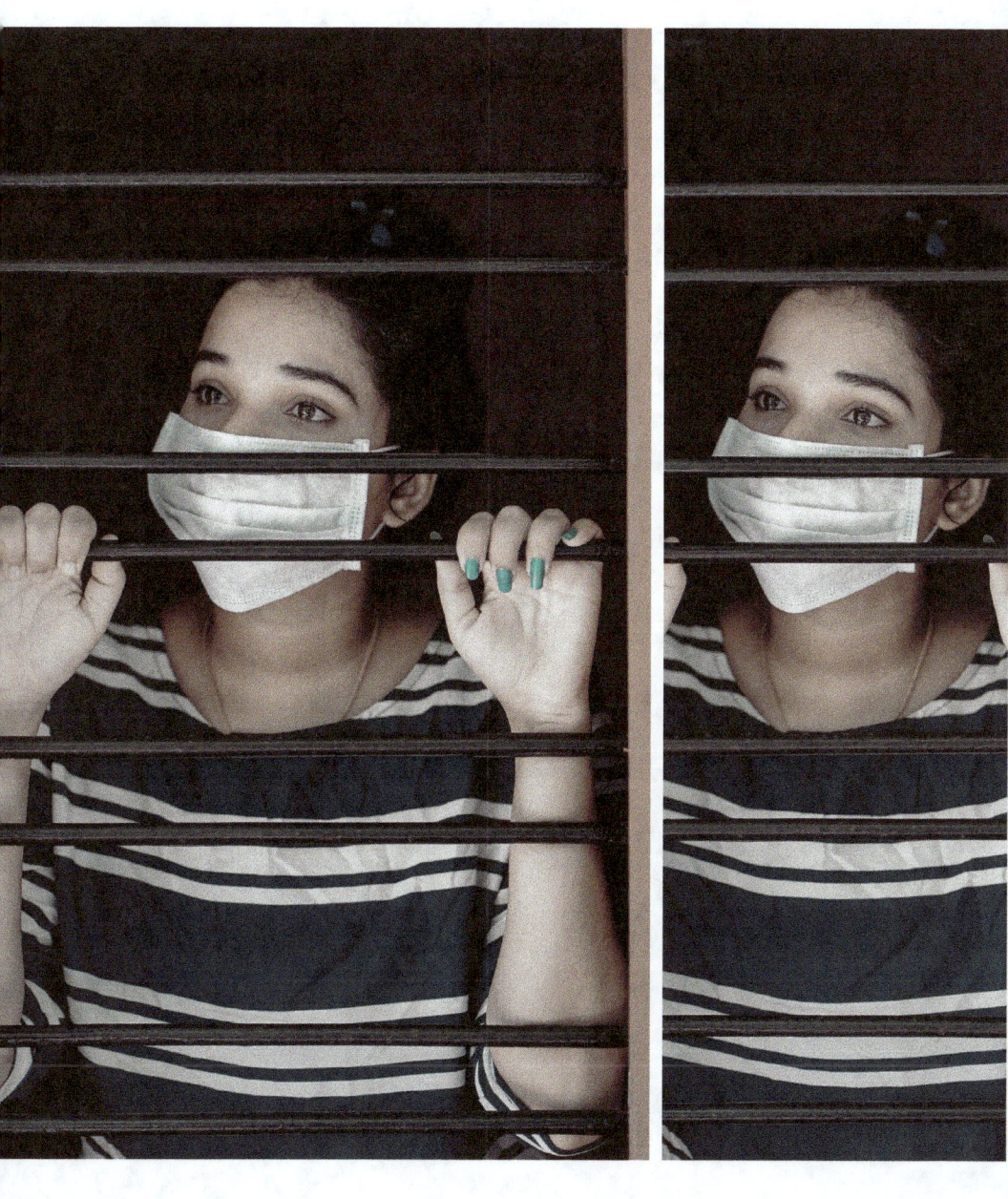

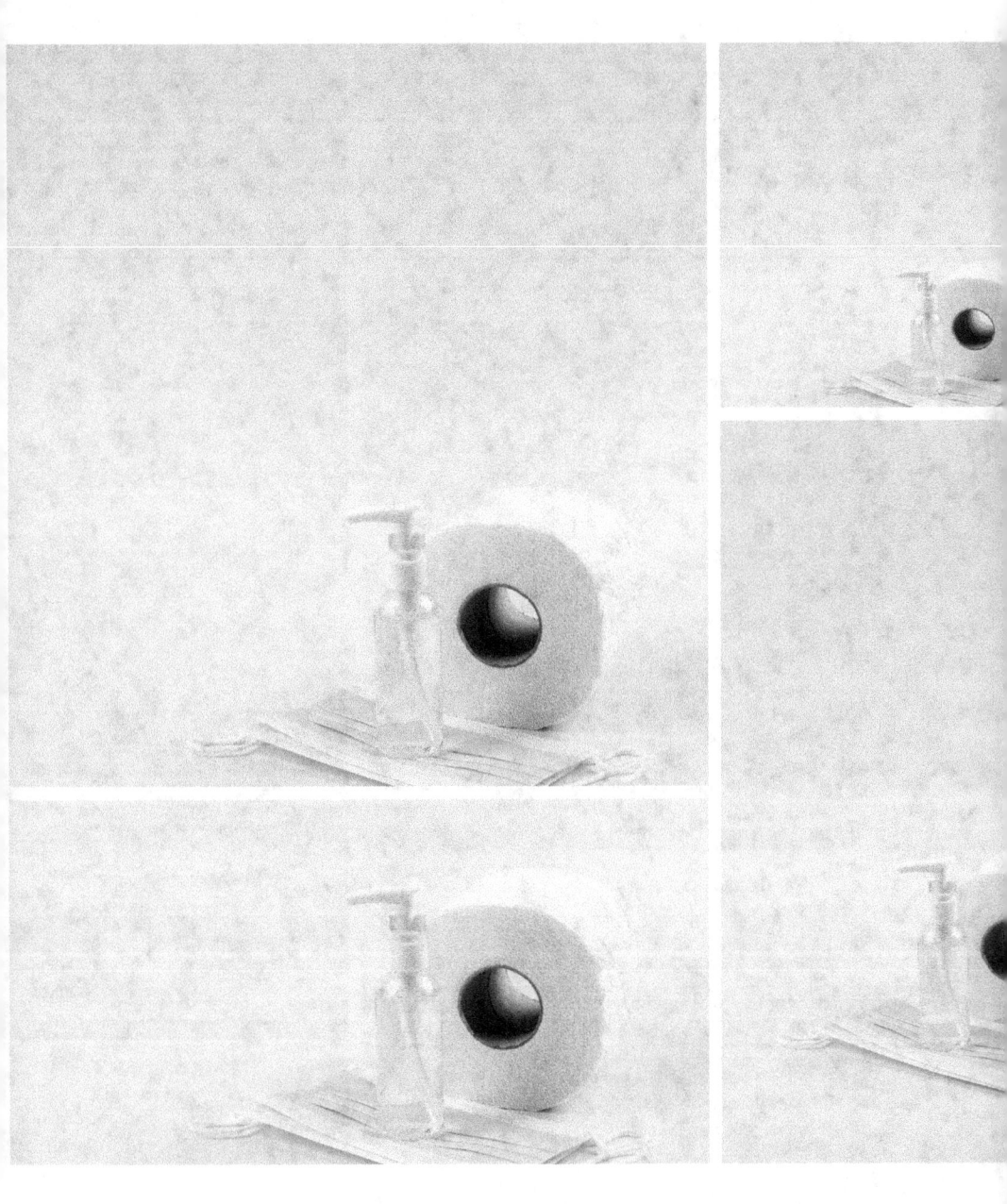

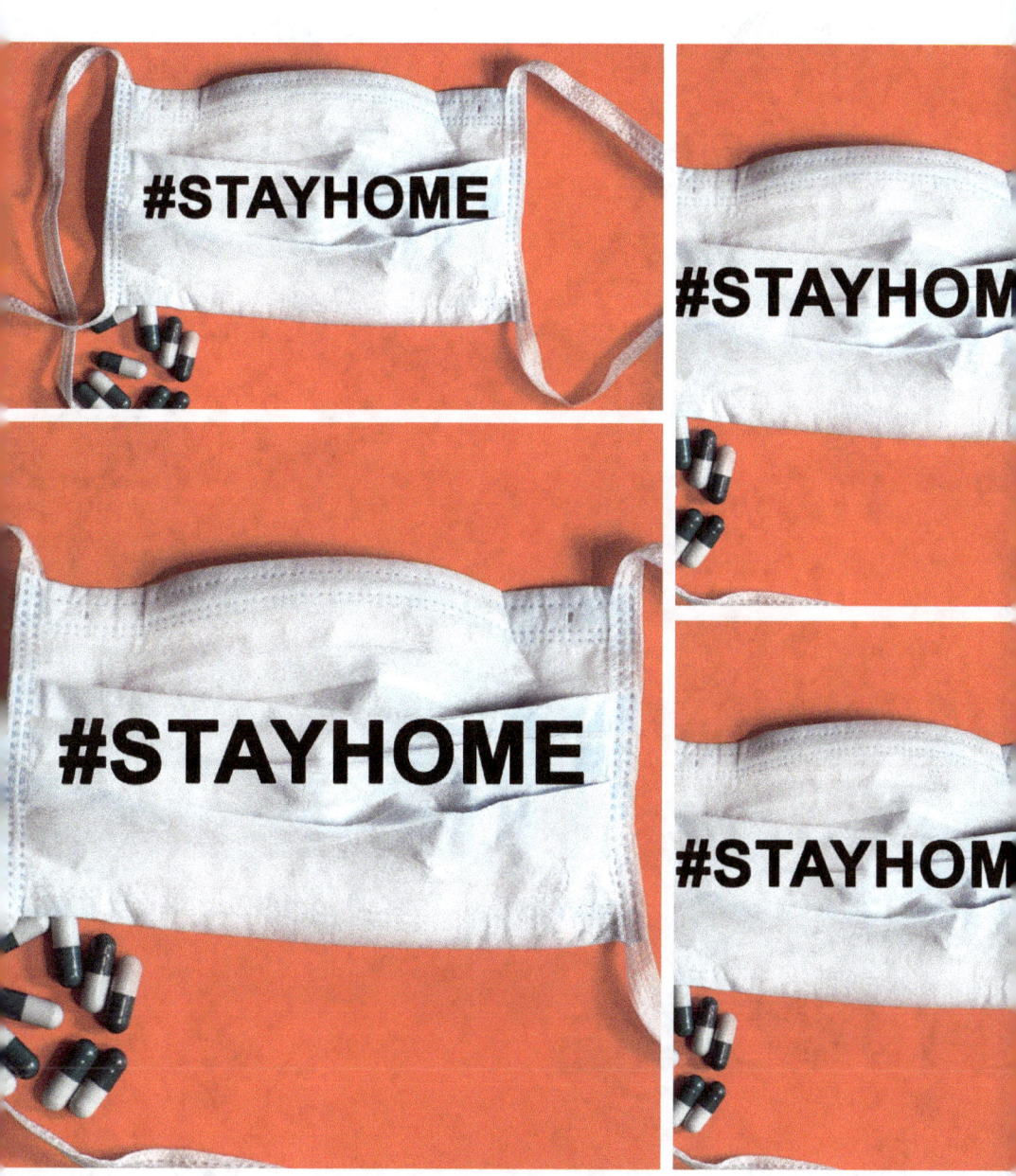

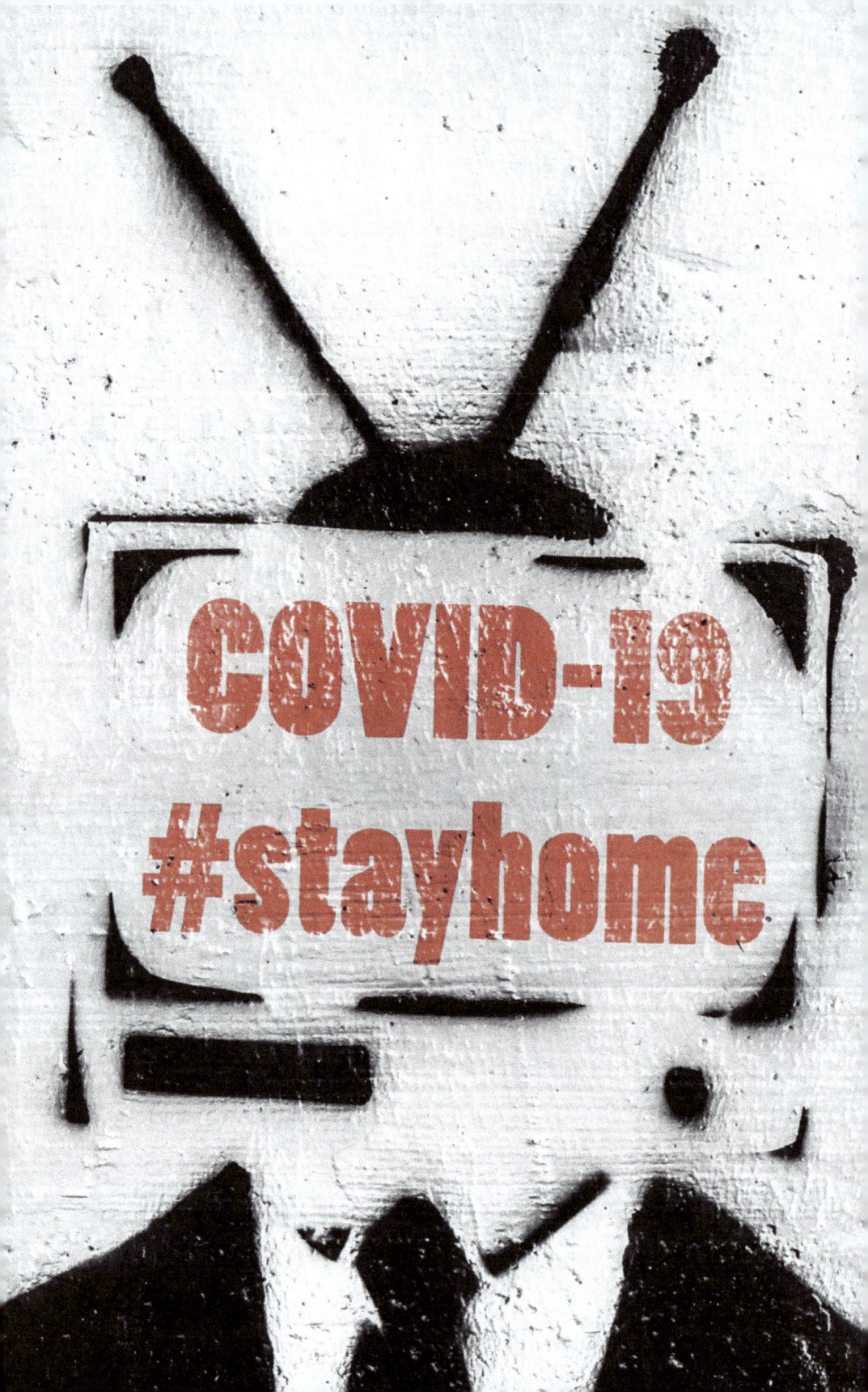

www.ingramcontent.com/pod-product-compliance
Lightning Source LLC
Chambersburg PA
CBHW070504220526
45467CB00002B/571